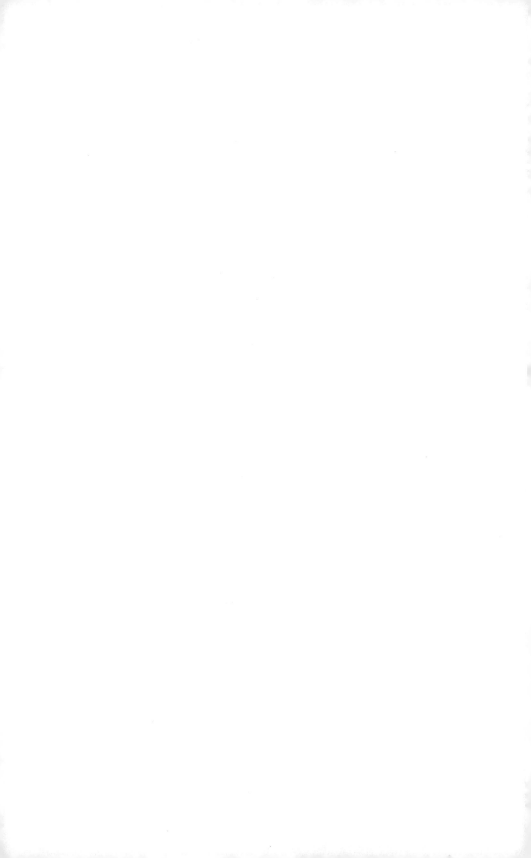

HOW TO SUCCEED IN THERAPY

HOW TO SUCCEED IN THERAPY

Navigating the Pitfalls on the Path to Wellness

Jared Scherz

ROWMAN & LITTLEFIELD
Lanham • Boulder • New York • London

Published by Rowman & Littlefield
A wholly owned subsidiary of The Rowman & Littlefield Publishing Group, Inc.
4501 Forbes Boulevard, Suite 200, Lanham, Maryland 20706
www.rowman.com

Unit A, Whitacre Mews, 26-34 Stannary Street, London SE11 4AB

British Library Cataloguing in Publication Information Available

Library of Congress Cataloging-in-Publication Data

Scherz, Jared.
How to succeed in therapy : Navigating the pitfalls on the path to wellness / by Jared Scherz.
pages cm.
Includes bibliographical references and index.
ISBN 978-1-4422-4134-3 (cloth : alk. paper) -- ISBN 978-1-4422-4135-0 (electronic)
1. Psychotherapy. 2. Psychotherapist and patient--Miscellana. I. Title.
RC475.S34 2015
616.89'14--dc23
2014030456

Printed in the United States of America

CONTENTS

PROJECTS BY AUTHOR

For all those people who either can't afford therapy, can't find a practitioner in your area who you are confident working with, or aren't ready to commit to the process, I am in the middle of developing a library of life lessons through a range of media such as video to help with your personal growth journey. You can find this emerging project at either www.itc-home.com or the ultimate home at www.txhelper.com.

For any clinician, coach, counselor, psychologist, motivational speaker, consultant, educator, physician, or personal growth advocate, I have created software that will help you bring your valuable lessons to people across the world. Through PsychPro software (www.psychpro.com), you can create your own self-help multimedia library for your own clients as well as those beyond your physical reach.

For educators who want coaching or personal/professional growth work, please visit TeacherCoach (www.teachercoach.com), where the specific needs of educators are being addressed to improve the lives of this most important profession.

Dr. Scherz is the author of other books, mainly related to schools and violence prevention. A list of these works includes:
Harnessing the Power of Resistance: A Guide for Educators
http://www.routledge.com/books/details/9781930556768/

The Truth about School Violence
   https://rowman.com/ISBN/9781578864560

Catastrophic School Violence: A New Approach to Prevention
   https://rowman.com/ISBN/9781610489850

Workbook for Preventing Catastrophic School Violence
   https://rowman.com/ISBN/9781475812428

It Can't Happen Here: One School Learns from Tragedy
   https://www.wavecloud.com/book/it-can-t-happen-here/978-1-62217-
158-3/12732476

ABOUT THE AUTHOR

Jared Scherz, PhD, has been working as a psychotherapist for over twenty years with individuals of all ages, issues, ethnicities, genders, and cultures, and focuses on both couples and group therapy. While trained in a variety of approaches, Scherz eventually found his home in gestalt therapy, where the client and therapist partner as a team to explore, understand, and experiment with the client's unfolding experience.

Scherz is the author of five published books in the field of education: *Harnessing the Power of Resistance*, *The Truth about School Violence*, *Catastrophic School Violence*, *Workbook for Preventing Catastrophic School Violence*, and *It Can't Happen Here*. He has an unpublished manuscript on couples therapy and has begun two new ventures including a social media networking site called ufeud (www.ufeud.com), where people are helped to navigate differences more productively.

In 2001, Scherz created the first wholeness center in New Jersey, called Integrated Therapy Center (ITC). The vision for ITC is to provide individuals with a wide range of holistic services such as yoga, nutrition, massage, psychoeducation, and physical conditioning to help in transforming the body, mind, and spirit. The center has a dual purpose of providing parallel types of services to small and large systems. The center is located in south central New Jersey.

He believes the focus of therapy is to empower the client or system toward recognition or awareness of both barriers toward improved health and inherent strengths within/between. He believes that goodness is inherent in every person, yet they hold themselves back in some shape or form or are held back by forces outside their control. He helps clients appreciate that change is paradoxical, in that a greater understanding of what keeps a person feeling stuck is needed before growth can occur. The broad goals of therapy are to help clients appreciate who they are, limitations and all, while recognizing and striving toward their full potential. This may mean finding closure with unfinished business from the past or learning how our experiences shape our present. Each person and/or system becomes more whole or integrated in order to function optimally.

He is also the creator of PsychPro (www.psychpro.com), a learning management software where helping professionals use a multimedia platform to enhance their practice. His next project, currently under way, is TxHelper (www.txhelper.com), where providers of health care are brought together with those seeking help in an online library of video courses to improve our health.

Scherz is also the founder of TeacherCoach (www.teachercoach.com), a site dedicated to improving the lives of educators. This project consists of bringing educators together to help build support and success around both personal growth and professional development goals.

Scherz is married to Donna Scherz, also a clinical psychologist. Together they live in Mount Laurel, New Jersey, with their three children, Cassidy (ten), Sera (nine), and Emma (seven), as well as their cat, Scarlett. At home Scherz is best known as Daddy, the gardener and chef, dedicated to raising a healthy and happy family.

USING THIS BOOK

This book is intended for people who are considering initiating self-discovery or personal growth work or have made the decision to start therapy, need guidance in what to expect/how to prepare, or are questioning whether their therapy is working optimally for them or if other approaches to wellness will suit them. Of the millions of people who seek therapy and other health-care services every day, only a fraction comprehend the full potential of therapy, which for the purpose of this book means personal growth work.

If you are onsidering therapy for the first time, or trying to improve upon a prior experience, you are not alone by far. More resources are available to people now than there were ten years ago, but there are few comprehensive guides, such as this one, that can help take you through the process from start to finish.

For those of you who have tried therapy and didn't feel successful, this book may help you understand what went "wrong" or what may need to be different this next time around. Maybe it was timing. The right therapy at the wrong time may still turn out poorly. Many people seek therapy in times of crisis but aren't yet ready to do the more involved work necessary to get to a higher level of health; instead, they aim to get through the initial crisis or to feel better quickly.

Or did you find a therapist you didn't click with and assumed that therapy just wasn't right for you? In some cases it's the client who isn't well prepared for therapy, and in other instances it's the therapist trying to fit his approach or style without adapting to what works best for you. A worthwhile therapist will be eager to explore this with you, looking at his role as well as encouraging you to examine your own.

I receive upwards of ten calls a week from new clients, many of whom have tried therapy before and didn't feel successful. Instead of laying blame, I inquire about previous therapy to get a sense of what did and didn't work for them. Could it simply have been a matter of gender—you really wanted a female therapist but only a male was available? Did you want someone who was going to be gentler instead of pushing you too fast? This is all good data for anyone who has made the attempt at therapy and is now ready to try again.

For those of you who are new to therapy, the opportunity exists to find a good match early on so that your first experience in therapy can be your last one. Some people will work with the same therapist on and off throughout their entire lives. Sometimes we make changes to get a new perspective even when the fit is a good one.

Each chapter in this book is designed to answer the most relevant and poignant questions of new clients and to provoke inquiry into how well your current therapy may be working for you. There is no order that these chapters need to be read in, and it's quite alright to skim different sections that seem important to you at the time. As any emerging field requires, feedback about how to improve the book for new readers is highly welcomed.

INTRODUCTION

A female client I recently worked with discontinued therapy before reaching any of her established goals. If asked, she would likely say that therapy was a "failed experience." She felt skeptical and highly cautious when she entered therapy with me. Her first experience with therapy was with a different psychologist with whom she felt she had become friends. As a result, she didn't experience the growth she thought she might have through counseling. If it weren't for her urgent need to relieve suffering, she might not ever have tried therapy again.

Following some early risk taking, which led to her feeling intensely vulnerable (to the point of being distressed), she found hope in the notion that she could potentially learn to trust again. Trust meant feeling exposed, which if history was any indicator of future events, would lead to further victimization. In spite of her fear, she began to recognize that old injuries were kept alive by not allowing herself to get close to people in the present. She learned it was okay to feel anger and even disgust with those who hurt her. This brilliant woman, who was tremendously successful at her career, spent very little time taking care of her own needs. Helping others was what gave her meaning, and it was safe because there was little risk on her part of rejection.

Less than ten sessions into our therapy, I observed to her that she did not appear to be having her therapy needs met. I suggested she may be primarily relating her experiences and feelings to me through her intellect, with compassion flowing only outward but not inward. This cautious approach to relating may have protected her from revealing too much of herself or being let down by others. I contrasted this approach with what I have come to understand as a deeper, more meaningful method of making contact that meets my needs as well as the other's simultaneously.

Instead of receiving my feedback as testament to her depth and potential for more fulfilling relationships, she heard it as criticism and bragging about my own evolution. It wasn't until later in the week that she shared this with me and shared her intention to discontinue therapy. I was incredulous about her reaction, as I'd had no intention of denigrating her or building myself up, but this is what she experienced. I attempted not to blame her for the misperception, because every person's reaction is important information. Instead, I tried to accept what she took from my input as a learning experience.

Regardless of what my intention was, it was unhelpful. More than that, it led to an experience that likely added to her distress and possibly sabotaged future therapy. While this is the very worst outcome a therapist and client can have, it can still be a learning experience if both look inward to decide what went wrong and what could have been done differently. Unfortunately, not enough people do this with failed attempts at therapy or events in their life.

In my twenty-five years of practice, I have spoken to many people who have tried therapy with another practitioner, reporting a very poor experience. I've heard complaints ranging from "all I kept getting was advice," "the person was so judgmental that I felt uncomfortable," "the clinician wanted to talk more about themselves than my issues," "they didn't seem qualified to help."

It's disturbing to hear of so many consistently dissatisfying experiences in therapy, leaving me worrying for all those people who will never try therapy a second time. Whether we are engaging in personal growth work, dealing with a crisis, or trying to address some important issue in our lives, therapy needs to be at a minimum safe and nonharmful. At its best, therapy becomes a transformational experience that takes us from surviving to thriving, recognizing that deep fulfillment is entirely possible.

For those of you who have tried therapy and not felt successful or are considering therapy or some other form of personal growth work, the goal is to optimize your energy into greater productivity. Too many people with good intentions aren't successful in this journey, and many lose the motivation to try again. Over ten million people, more than 4 percent of the nation's population, have met with a mental health professional, but over 30 percent stopped after one or two sessions, indicating they were either poorly prepared or didn't find the right fit with their therapist. [1]

More than half of the general adult population believes that it is somewhat or very difficult to access mental health treatment, and 37 percent of all insured respondents in one study were unsure of whether their health insurance covered mental health care. Therapy is too important for people to endure poor fits or avoid treatment altogether because they are unsure how to proceed.

"When it comes to selecting a therapist—a choice that represents a substantial investment of time and money—people often exercise as little personal preference as they do when hailing a taxi cab," says Jo Colman, CEO of *Psychology Today*. But how do we sift through the abundance of information to make this difficult but important decision?

If your car is having engine problems, you might go to the nearest mechanic in your neighborhood, hoping not to get ripped off. If you are pregnant and needing a pediatrician, you may ask your friends and family for a referral to a doctor they know. In both examples we hope the professional we find is going to have expertise in their field, enough integrity so we can trust them, and if we are lucky a comfort level that makes working with them pleasurable.

We don't ask the mechanic for a résumé or recommendations from former customers, assuming their being in business means they are reputable. We attribute value to the mere notion that they are available and interested in serving us, regardless of whether they may be the best choice. For professionals such as the pediatrician, we may add a further assumption that they went to school and received their MD, meaning they are fully qualified to treat our child.

In some instances, we may return to somebody who has done work for us even if we weren't completely satisfied. We do this by adjusting our expectations to fit the results, sometimes for convenience but other times because we hold doubt that making a change will yield better results.

Taking this approach is risky when trying to find a therapist or healthcare provider. At a time when we may be feeling vulnerable, overwhelmed, or even desperate to change something in our lives, we may accept the first opportunity for help that presents itself. You can find your mechanic abrasive, but if he fixes your car, you may be satisfied. Even a surgeon with a lousy bedside manner will be tolerated if he operates successfully. But skill level alone is only one determining factor for a therapist.

Finding the right approach to health care is both a personal and a professional choice and one that presents more barriers than other sought-out services. Firstly, we may not feel comfortable asking somebody for a referral, which is often how we find professionals in our community. Secondly, we may not know what questions to ask or what to be on the lookout for. We can't ask for recommendations because of privacy, so we are left without a clear idea of how to make this most important choice.

If this initial layer of difficulty isn't challenging enough, add in the complexities of managed care (health insurance), the hundreds of different styles and philosophies therapists work from, and the nuances of how someone seems to you when you first speak with them, and it can be quite discouraging. Due to all these impediments, we often make decisions based on convenience, availability, and affordability, keeping our fingers crossed that whomever we choose is going to be the best choice.

Leaving this up to chance will sometimes result in a good fit but may always leave a person wondering if they would be better served with somebody else. Learning how to listen to one's gut can be helpful in this regard, because our brain is oftentimes advocating based on pragmatics. For instance, your brain may tell you, "the therapist is close to my home," "they take my insurance," and "she was the only female psychologist available." Our brains can and will overshadow our gut feeling, especially when we don't have anything to compare it with.

Clients who tried therapy and weren't pleased will often say that they didn't realize it could have been different. Not trusting oneself or having the appropriate expectations can lead people to waste valuable time and money, or worse, leave therapy feeling discouraged, believing they aren't fixable or this is as good as it gets. This book is about knowing when the therapist isn't the best one for the job and making the best choice to start with.

Just like in any other field, there are some truly gifted therapists—inspirations to others—but there are also some very ineffective therapists. And yet sometimes even the very best therapist may not be the right therapist for you in your particular situation with your set of needs and goals. When you are feeling desperate and vulnerable, it is difficult to be discriminating about finding the therapist who is best suited to work with you, since you may lack the energy and focus to make a clear decision.

You may be lacking hope in general, so your temptation is to rush getting started.

Urgency and outright desperation can lead you to make an impulsive decision you may later regret. Putting a little bit more energy into the screening and preparation process can make a world of difference in your therapeutic journey. In this book, I have provided a clear outline of important issues to consider, questions to ask, and obstacles to anticipate so that you can learn to get your needs met.

And lastly you will want to recognize that everything being brought to your attention may vary greatly based on individual preferences. Try to be mindful that character traits and other dynamics being pointed out are appealing to you for particular reasons of possible import, and consider what that is about. If you don't need somebody who is warm but instead seek out somebody who is more clinical, what is this telling you about yourself? The process for finding a therapist can be the start to your personal growth journey if approached with a sense of curiosity.

Even if we decide to discontinue therapy, try to have an ending that supports a healthy new beginning. Mistakes or mishaps are only unfortunate if nothing is learned. I hope this book helps you take a new look at personal growth work so obstacles are turned into important growth opportunities.

I

Understanding Psychotherapy

My Light

A life of pain and relentless torture
The only light, a train headed my way.
Relief seemed impossible, that doesn't happen for me.
Never knowing how I will survive the day.
I can't run away from it forever.
Growing tired, pain won't relent.
A place for my burdens to unveil.
A safe base, no further descent.
Through therapy, we create a path.
I can't do it alone; I simply can't cope.
A team is created, fears slowly abate;
No longer alone, I breathe in new hope.
We trudge our way through my darkness;
The train, growing its light.
The wounds revealed, we move at my pace;
With unrelenting support, we carve out my plight.
I see no train, but the light remains;
A glimmer, a sparkle ahead.
The light of freedom and peace I squint to see.
A light I no longer dread.
To live a life void of intense fear and shame;
The gift of my therapist by my side.

My goal, to continue towards the light
With healed scars no longer I hide.

Maria A

I

WHAT IS (PSYCHO) THERAPY?

THERAPY DEFINED

Therapy comes from the root word *therapeutic*, meaning "to treat or heal." There are many types of therapy, including physical, occupational, recreational, speech, and drug therapies such as those used to treat cancer. In this book we use the term *therapy* as an abbreviation of another specific type called *psychotherapy*, or professional help to improve mental health or psychological functioning (relational, behavioral, existential, experiential, phenomenological, emotional, etc.).

We are always in a state of becoming; thus, change is constant. Some changes are intentional, and other changes go on outside our awareness. Aging, for instance, alters the composition of our bodies, first building tissue and then decaying it. Learning creates new neuropathways in our brain; socializing expands and contracts our network of support; and living offers opportunities every day for financial, medical, recreational, and countless other areas of expansion/contraction, broadening, and narrowing in our lives.

With this ongoing change process, we are simultaneously dealing with another equally powerful dynamic, and that is the force for sameness. Sameness is like earth's gravity, preventing us from running, climbing, and jumping too high or too fast. The force for sameness or persistence helps us from experiencing chaos that accompanies too much change too quickly, feeling out of control. Oftentimes, life unfolds in a way that seems outside our sphere of influence, and in response we may slam on the brakes to avoid feeling swept away like a small sailboat in a typhoon.

The balance between the forces for sameness and change produces a tension that pressurizes the body. Depending on how the strands of our personhood are intertwined, this tug-of-war may break down these existential fibers that hold us together. If we have been through recent or chronic distress, if we are feeling especially fragile, or if our network of support is compromised, we may experience this tension between sameness and change as a threat to our being, our wholeness.

As we begin to feel pulled apart, sometimes outside of our awareness, we dis-integrate or fragment into parts. In an effort to keep the ship righted through the storm we may emphasize those parts of ourselves that are most pleasing or comfortable or that seem safest. Therapy, in its simplest form, is a place to work on preventing further breakdown of these connective fibers while building new ones, helping us to feel more whole again. Therapy helps us deal with the forces for sameness and change so that we become excited about the prospects for growth as opposed to fearful about the outcomes.

Sometimes therapy is about altering the way we respond to this distress so that we feel more intact, and sometimes it's about becoming more accepting of what is outside our control—coming to terms with what is and what has been. Whether you are looking for symptom relief such as alleviation of anxiety or depression, seeking out closure on unfinished business from the past, or embarking on a transformative journey to find more fulfillment in life, therapy can be a powerful medium to reach toward your goals. The short-term, solution-focused approach and the longer-term self-discovery process both offer a reliable and supportive partnership to reach your objectives. The methods of doing so, however, can vary widely according to your wants and the therapist's orientation, as will be described in greater detail later.

While psychotherapy is considered to be taking place when a professional clinician and a client meet, this doesn't always occur inside an office. Many activities can be therapeutic: exercising, taking walks, hitting balls in a batting cage, going to a comedy club, or anything else that creates energy or space for catharsis, self-awareness, or personal growth.

Some therapists help through more conventional means like the ones shown on television programs and movies. Other therapists partake more actively in this journey. A therapist who is helping a client with a fear of closed spaces, for instance, may plan trips outside the office to help with in-vivo exposure to the "aversive stimulus." Even more simply, a therapist may take a young child outside for a walk to build trust and comfort.

Therapy is an active process that continues during the course of your week, in between appointments and off the proverbial "couch." What is being learned or considered is applied at home, at work, out with friends, or at any other event in which you experience some significant form of tension. While this book doesn't fully explore the therapeutic work done outside the office, the important message here is that therapy doesn't end when the session is over.

Therapy is a creative process that can be formal and traditional, yet it can also be spontaneous, inventive, and daring. The restrictions placed on therapy are set forth by the participants yet adaptable to the unique needs of each individual. Prescriptive approaches that emphasize a certain mode of operations may be comforting to some who want structure and rigid to those who need more freedom. Sometimes what is needed by a client isn't what is the most helpful to them, so keep in mind what your tendencies are and be willing to lean into your discomfort.

THE MAIN COMPONENTS OF THERAPY

*A **partnership** is an alliance between two or more people with the aim of achieving a common goal or set of goals.* The first step is coming to agree upon both the nature of the partnership and the anticipated outcome of the relationship/work together. The therapist investigates what the client expects of themselves/the therapist and conversely, the therapist may share his or her expectations, wants, and wishes for the client. Clarifying both positions helps reduce the potential for unnecessary complications distracting from the work.

Some therapists believe that any divergence in perspectives is grist for the mill and ought to be looked upon as an opportunity to learn. For instance, what happens if the client doesn't give a twenty-four-hour notice before canceling an appointment and the therapist expects to be compensated for his or her time? What happens if a client attempts to contact the therapist in an emergency but can't get through because the therapist is working with other clients during the day? Establishing some ground rules at the onset of therapy is a helpful way to avoid these complications, but talking through what is elicited through these disappointments, perceived rejections, and hurts can be illuminating.

A therapist may provide a disclaimer or statement of understanding form prior to the first session for this very purpose. Such a document is an agreement of sorts, similar to other business arrangements, including legal descriptions of privacy. This may seem formal and rigid; however, it is required of most professionals by law, their governing and regulating bodies (such as the American Psychological Association and American Counseling Association), malpractice insurance, the insurance companies with whom they hold contracts, and HIPPA (Health Insurance Portability and Accountability Act).

A contract also helps to address the inherent power differential which exists or is perceived to exist in therapy. While this relationship is referred to as a partnership, know that some therapists view themselves in the expert role, creating an automatic disparity of power. In traditional psychoanalysis, for example, the client lies on a couch with the therapist or analyst interpreting his or her unconscious, thereby creating another type of power imbalance. Reactions to the therapist in this orientation are often considered projections and not true relational issues to be worked through. A partnership therefore is not necessarily 50/50 in the eyes of all therapists and orientations.

A power differential may be experienced between client and therapist, depending upon two things: the first is how the client views the therapist, and the second is the attitude and belief system of the therapist. A client may feel comforted by putting the therapist in the expert role and may look toward them for advice and/or direction. The therapist may also see themselves in the expert role, not viewing the relationship as a partnership to be explored.

Even the terms used to describe a consumer of therapy have changed for many theoretical orientations, signaling that shift in power. Most recently, the therapist-client relationship (further evidenced by a shift in language from "patient" to "client") is viewed as more balanced. Clients may still want to defer to the professional for expert guidance; however, most therapists tend to shy away from this role, viewing it as creating dependence and not interdependence. The process of building a client's self-support and resiliency is termed *empowerment*, which will be discussed in later chapters.

As in any well-designed partnership, the participants will prepare for the inevitable disagreements, hurts, and other conflicts that are both anticipated and unexpected. Differences are not just likely, they are desirable. Differences are a way to help broaden perspectives and better negotiate for what one needs.

A skilled clinician will welcome discussion around differences, helping you to feel understood and valued in your disagreement. They will also help you attend to how you differ. Do you swallow what is given to you whole without chewing, or do you disregard what is offered without much consideration? Differences will exist from the very beginning of therapy, when goals are being discussed, through the end point of deciding when to terminate.

No rule says that therapist and client have to agree on the "what" or the "how" of things. A helpful therapist will listen to and respect the desired aims of his or her client while offering input about related areas of potential help. For instance, a new client tells her therapist she wants to learn how to "cope better" with her stressful job. The therapist may come to believe that the job is creating so much adversity that remaining in the position is detrimental to the person's health. Does the therapist respect the client's wishes or promote a different agenda?

Some believe the therapist's beliefs or biases have no place in therapy, while others use their self-experience to guide them in their helping. While advice is not generally considered a deep and meaningful therapeutic tool, it's inevitable that suggestions will occur in some shape or form. Gestalt therapy may be an exception, as the therapist intends to share their experience of the client above their thought or opinion, helping elucidate the client's own discoveries.

*Therapy requires a **method** of gaining insight, awareness, or understanding about what is hidden or unknown to us. Through this process of making the hidden seen, we better appreciate our attributes and limitations that influence our approach to situations, events, or relatedness.*

Therapists have a job parallel to that of teachers, but more subtle and loosely defined. Therapists have no curriculum or syllabus other than a philosophy of change and perhaps the steps to accomplish certain objectives. Therapists do, however, advocate for looking both inwardly or outwardly to expand our sometimes-narrow perspective, seeking information to help in our growth.

With more input from the outside and awareness from within, we can better understand how we have become stuck. Whether we haven't healed from the past, created harmony in a current relationship, or found satisfaction in who we are or what we do, we need to understand the dilemma before we can change it. A therapist's job is to help find avenues to generate this new information.

Some therapists bypass this part of the process, believing change is the important element. They believe that once a person experiences the benefit of doing something differently, he will gain the needed energy to overcome obstacles. This is true for some people who haven't felt success in a long time or who need to experience newness to open new doorways. For others where resistance to change is too high, a slower discovery process may be needed. It isn't easy to ask for the therapist to take his time during that initial call, but it's important if you are going to learn to ask for what you need.

Polarities is a concept that can help in either approach. If we use the idea of polarities, we come to appreciate how our approach or viewpoint is neither good nor bad, but skewed toward the end of a particular continuum, the result of which are disadvantages we may not have been aware of. Through the lens of polarities we are better able to see what is hidden to us, avoiding the pitfalls of labeling or pathologizing (using diagnostic labels to categorize and define dysfunction).

Everything works on a continuum between two polarities. We aren't strong or frail, adventurous or conservative, open or closed, expressive or withdrawn, but somewhere in between, depending upon how we measure ourselves. Moving away from good/bad, positive/negative, right/wrong, we begin to appreciate benefits and limitations of every aspect of who we are and how we work. Removing the judgment from our perspective allows us to gain a greater understanding of who we are.

We can often find pluses and minuses to actions and events that make choosing a path difficult. We can take the day off from work to rebuild our energy, but if we do so we may return the next day with more work piled up. Without clear good and bad it may seem like choices become more complex, and in a sense this is true. It requires we let go of outcomes and be more appreciative of the processes by which we arrive at decisions.

*Therapy requires a **process** by which we examine differences between who we are and who we want to be, how we go about getting our needs* *met, and how we make use of the resources available to us. This helps us become less outcome focused.*

Therapy is a place to explore one's existence. We may seek to answer the existential questions of Who am I? What am I? How do I matter? And how does all this compare with what I hold as the ideal? These philosophical questions are joined by more concrete ones, including Why do I continue to encounter this same problem or experience this same symptom? Through ongoing dialogue, introspection, and feedback, therapist and client put together the pieces of a puzzle that form the picture of our life.

Understanding *what is* helps us to appreciate what it may take to create something different. This exploration of what currently exists will likely involve all the systemic influences on a person—such as community, culture, religion, work, family, friendships—and other more contextual factors such as finances, health, and geography. Because we do not exist in a vacuum, we become curious about how all these influences have guided us toward particular decisions and shaped how we fit into the world.

There Are No Children Here is a book written by Alex Kotlowitz,[1] depicting the life of two African American boys growing up in the projects of inner-city Chicago. The boys resort to stealing, fighting, and forms of survival not because it's who they want to be but because it's what they believe they need to exist. We may expect these boys, as adults, to have trouble with trust and perhaps intimacy because they have been conditioned to attend to more basic needs.

In therapy, they may assess how well the coping mechanisms learned early in life are working for them currently. They may feel safe, for instance, if they keep others at a distance, but at what cost to their need for belonging? Some adults who have experienced trauma early in life tend toward greater caution in their adulthood, while others may go in the direction of risky behavior, even disregarding their own health. Neither response is good or bad, but these learned tendencies may no longer be effective for the adult.

Trauma survivors may have difficulty asking for and negotiating getting their needs met because it doesn't feel safe. Others, who were fortunate enough to avoid such a blatant disregard for boundaries, may still have difficulty meeting their needs because they learned less adaptive strategies growing up. A scary but powerful way of improving in this way is through group therapy, discussed in a later chapter. A process group mirrors more experiential therapies that help us emphasize "how" over "what."

Let's consider the process of reducing anxiety and stress. There is a tendency to want to "stop stressing" or be calm. This focus on the outcome, rather than on the process by which we achieve this goal, can actually increase tension. It may not seem evident, but we have far less control over how things turn out than we do over how we address them. This is an important shift to begin reducing anxiety. By shifting our focus to our own processes, we are helped to identify patterns, cycles, and other repetitive behaviors that slow down our movement toward greater health.

Along the same lines, helpful therapists are surprisingly *less* interested in content. Situations, events, circumstances, and all the other contextual elements of your life are exceedingly tempting to share with your therapist. After all, if he or she doesn't know what's going on, how can they be helpful, right? The opposite may be true in many instances. Your therapist may be doing you disservice if they focus exclusively on content, because the risk of overlooking themes that come from *how* we do things is greater.

This doesn't mean that data isn't important. Painting a picture for a therapist may help you feel better, knowing you have described sometimes complex and traumatizing events from your life. Sometimes details of your predicament lend valuable clues to the patterns identified earlier, so long as each session isn't simply a strategizing meeting where advice and solutions are offered.

*Therapy requires an **appreciation** of who we are and what aspects of ourselves need to be accepted as opposed to changed. Until we can appreciate who we are and what we have experienced, we cannot move from surviving to thriving.*

Sometimes therapy isn't about changing but learning how to be more accepting of who and what we are. For some therapists, self-acceptance is an overarching goal of all therapy. For example, if a woman tells her therapist she wants to become more assertive, she may be helped to find barriers that inhibit her self-expression, while also trying to appreciate her softness. Being confluent (a merging of boundaries so there is no clear sense of self) can lead to being taken advantage of, but it may also mean being flexible and sensitive to the needs of others. The therapist works with her to understand how she suppresses her voice while learning to deal with the fears of making herself heard, all the while appreciating the inherent value in who she already is.

Pigs Eat Wolves is a wonderful book written by Charles Bates.[2] Through the fairy tale of the Three Little Pigs, the author helps us understand how we disconnect from aspects of our personhood we do not like and/or are not comfortable with. The wolf represents all of these unwanted and detached pieces of ourselves that we project onto the world, causing us to externalize fears and diminish our sense of control (safety). The pig at first erects a primitive house made of sticks, moving on to more complex structures such as brick to keep the wolf at bay; in the same way, a person is still fragmented but has more sophisticated protective mechanisms guarding him or her from intimacy. Ultimately, the author teaches us that the way to wholeness is to swallow the wolf or accept that which we most fear.

There is an old saying describing our tendency to take back our own problems when we see them in a pile with everybody else's. This same idea holds true for things we don't like about ourselves such as traits, experiences, conflicts, and characteristics. It doesn't mean we don't want to be thinner, stronger, smarter, or more athletic. It means that we are a product of all of our "stuff," and over time we learn to grow more comfortable with who we are. Not only does this predictability allow us to face life with greater certainty in the wake of constant change, it helps us to come to terms with who we are.

Appreciating who we are, frailties and all, requires a few things first. We need to feel confident enough to identify and own those less desirable pieces, we need to feel hopeful that we are working toward self-improvement, and we need a context in which we don't feel judged but cared for, and not in spite of our inequities but because of them.

In addition to the unconditional positive regard (a facet of humanistic theory created by Carl Rogers) described above, clients need to have their ideas, thoughts, feelings, desires, needs, and actions validated. This does not connote agreement but recognition of the value or purpose for who we have become.[3] With some antiquated traits that don't serve us anymore, we want to appreciate how at one time they may have served us well. Cautiousness, for example, may have protected us as a child with a critical parent, but as an adult it may thwart intimacy.

Therapy requires **support** *through encouragement, challenge, and accountability for strategic risk taking. Therapy is a place to feel safe enough to explore while leaning on the edge of discomfort.*

People seeking therapy often feel alone, misunderstood, and unsupported. Relief from the burden of solitude is often the first priority in therapy. Unconditional positive regard means the therapist may not always like or agree with what their clients are saying or doing, but they always accept them as people without judgment and with unconditional positive regard.[4]

This doesn't mean that therapists are disingenuous. Without being authentic, there can be no trust and no conflict to work through (constructive exploration of differences). Therapy is about a balance of trust and discomfort, where we feel valued enough to become vulnerable. Through our vulnerability, we can explore what is generating our distress, using the support we feel in therapy to delve deeper into the issues.

Support does not mean agreement, and it doesn't have to include affirmation or encouragement. Gently confronting somebody about apparent incongruence can buttress one's awareness, which can be one of the most supportive experiences to have. If we care about somebody, we want them to know what we see that they may be missing, even if it's unpleasant to hear.

Sometimes support is a more literal translation, such as the supportive structures in a building that hold up beams. By holding clients accountable to their work, therapists also support their efforts that promote growth. A therapist may say, "I'm concerned you didn't follow through on your plan for healthier eating. I'm wondering what interfered with your desire to be more energized." Helping someone hold themselves accountable, raising the bar to one's own standards, can be tremendously supportive.

Replenishment *is integral when we feel depleted or even burned out. If we don't feel restored, we will lack the needed energy to self-examine, take risks, and feel well enough to make contact.*

Depleted energy is a common experience of clients entering therapy, especially when they have waited a long while to seek help. When we are putting out more than we are taking in—common for caregiver types and workaholics—then exhaustion can set in. Encouragement, reassurance, and caring may be helpful for the emotional refueling until a person learns how to develop better self-care strategies. Having forty-five minutes in which nothing is asked or expected of you other than being yourself is a way to recharge.

Reflective listening (helping a client to feel heard and understood by reframing or restating what is said) as a means of empathy is another common way therapists help their clients refuel. Being heard and seen is a powerful experience, especially when it isn't received from friends and family. Permission to be ourselves, being heard, and feeling cared for allows us to rebuild our energy reserves.

The most powerful of all methods to restore energy comes from making better contact within (the self) and between ourselves and others. Someone who is out of contact with his body may have forgotten how to attend to his senses, finding replenishment in reconnecting with those lost parts. This may simply mean eating a meal and paying attention to the sensations associated with hunger and satiation or taking a bath but using scented oils to help us breathe in greater relaxation.

When we develop greater internal awareness, we can generate energy that helps us to integrate our physical selves. The more distracted, spread out, and fragmented we are, the more diluted our energy becomes. Imagine the body as a series of lengthy circuits, any one of which can interrupt the flow of electricity when loose or disconnected.

Making better contact with others also helps build our energy stores. Meaningful exchanges filled with honesty, openness, and curiosity can help to stimulate us in a way we cannot do alone. Making better contact with the world can also generate energy, because we feel a part of the earth. Planting in a garden, feeling the sun on our head and the cool earth in our toes, uses the available resources around us to recharge.

Exploring the reasons for your diminishing energy stores is important for self-sustaining restoration. Sometimes we are faced with situations outside our control, such as injury and illness, the need to make money to survive, or rebuilding from catastrophic events, but the majority of people simply don't budget their energy well. As is the case with finances, we want to have a positive balance at the end of the day, which is often difficult to achieve. Even if we go to bed tired, we strive to be inspired, productive, and meaningful so that our energy is well spent. Similar to investing in high-interest-bearing accounts, we need to invest our energy wisely.

Creating and sustaining energy are two related but distinct tasks. If we are to continue setting and reinforcing limits with a pushy family member, for instance, we need both a reserve of energy and a constantly replenishing well to draw upon. Be aware, however, that ignoring or tolerating the pushy family member isn't conserving energy as we might believe. Holding on to or swallowing feelings is more draining than we realize. Imagine a ballerina standing on one leg, atop a balance beam, trying to remain still, holding her position so she keeps her muscles taut. Adjusting positions also requires energy and is sometimes why people choose to remain stuck in the same position, especially when the new position is unfamiliar and likely uncomfortable at first.

When we are struggling in our lives, energy is at a premium. Therapy helps us move away from conservation into more calculated risk-taking endeavors that generate successes. Building energy toward change is an important task of the therapist and client.

*A **search** for greater meaning and purpose in one's life is a component of therapy for those seeking more than symptom relief.*

The existential search for meaning (Why am I here? What is my purpose? What is the meaning of my life?) is necessary in finding greater fulfillment. Life is an ongoing journey layered with constant impediments. Self-actualization, as it's referred to by Abraham Maslow, reminds us that we have basic needs at the foundation of who we are (safety/security) but higher-order needs that lead us toward happiness. Climbing Maslow's hierarchy takes us further from corporal needs toward those that intersect with the world.[5]

Those who are depressed will resonate with the idea that their life seems pointless or lacks passion. Passion means waking up in the morning with excitement to face the day and satisfaction at day's end for making the most of your waking hours. This is the type of passion that many who exist on a day-to-day basis miss out on because they are struggling to exist.

Those who are anxious may realize they are outcome focused, living in the past or the future but not the present. What drives them is completion of tasks; they derive satisfaction from making check marks on their never ending to-do list. This approach to life resembles the hamster wheel, where lots of energy is expended to end up with only have-tos and few want-tos. Life is more exciting when the outcome isn't completely planned; however, it can be scary to adopt such a paradigm. Instead of a wheel, it's more like a never ending series of forks in the road, taking the less interesting-looking path. Therapy helps people garner the courage to seek out the unknown and take the road less traveled. To make this choice, one lives in the here and now, a concept addressed in more depth later.

Finding closure *with unfinished business from the past is important for many. As unresolved issues are worked through, we are able to free up energy while finding greater peace.*

Therapy involves some level of trust and comfort that allows us to recognize and then reduce our protectiveness. If we feel secure within therapy, we are more likely to acknowledge the shame, embarrassment, anger, and pain that we carry with us. Both the therapist and the client are responsible for building safety, and they do this through risk taking, honesty, and receptivity to bidirectional feedback. An open invitation for clients to safely say when they disagree, need to slow the pace, or want to take therapy in a different direction can help to build this trust.

A common mistake clients make is not telling therapists when they are dissatisfied, because holding back this information doesn't afford the therapist an opportunity to be more flexible in his approach or investigate the nature of the client's discomfort. Safety is an ongoing process that may wax and wane throughout the life of the therapy.

Many seek therapy to work through unpleasant and oftentimes painful experiences from their past. Child abuse, sexual molestation, severe neglect, violence, and other violations of one's personhood may result in trauma, creating emotional scars that we carry into our adulthood. Understanding the extent to which these incidents and experiences influence our current sense of self is a highly challenging but rewarding task of therapy.

Trauma is only one type of experience that leaves us feeling unresolved. Countless episodes or experiences in our lives don't get finished, either because we are too fearful, we decide not to expend the energy, or we don't realize they require more work. Each time we are hurt through the actions of another, we may choose to keep this feeling to ourselves, wanting to avoid appearing weak or vulnerable. A supervisor who influences our status within the organization, a parent who may withhold love and acceptance, or a friend who seems unreceptive to feedback are all examples of people with whom we may feel incomplete, because we have held back how we are feeling.

Unfinished business may be an intrapersonal experience, not involving others. Failing to qualify for the Olympics, deciding not to go to college, or not applying for a promotion at work can leave us feeling incomplete. In therapy, we seek to identify where these unresolved experiences exist, to what extent they impact our lives, and what can be done to find resolution. If we don't work on finding closure with this unfinished business, then it continues to influence us in our relationships and serves to create distress that we don't attend to. True acceptance only comes when we have worked through our feelings in an honest and open way.

*A **means of identifying barriers** that interfere with reaching your potential is needed to avoid roadblocks that inhibit your growth. Sometimes these barriers are external and need to be dealt with through life changes, but most times they are self-imposed.*

We all have the potential for greatness, but that greatness can be obscured or even curtailed when we are faced with unpleasantness. Whether our greatness is intended to help make a difference in the lives of others, achieve personal glory, or change the world in some significant way, we face both external and internal forces that hinder our efforts. Some of these obstacles are out of our control and require a change in approach, while others are self-generated.

Self-imposed barriers include fears of failure embedded in us from early in our lives or other forces for sameness. Therapy aims at uncovering these oftentimes hidden subtexts that are deeply rooted in our life scripts. Hypnosis, analysis, psychodrama, dream interpretation, and other techniques designed to shed light on these hard-to-see areas may be used to illuminate the obstacles. From insight to action, therapy intends to create new neuronal and behavioral pathways for growth.

In its simplest form, therapy is like having a personal trainer who can help you rehearse new ways of thinking, feeling, and behaving. Challenging you to stretch beyond your comfort zone, therapists assist in reaching beyond the parameters we have placed around our existence. Reaching your potential means working through all the impediments, often unrecognized, but highly limiting.

*An **environment** to experiment and rehearse new ways of thinking, relating, and being is created in therapy. Much like a laboratory used by scientists, the therapy office can be a place to test a hypothesis before implementing it in your everyday life.*

In this human laboratory the client is both the researcher and often the subject of the experiment. Sometimes the therapist plays the role of the subject, allowing the client to try out assertiveness, for instance, to see how it feels and what the reaction may be.

While a client may feel an increase in resistance to interpretation, many therapists use this strategy to point out what they believe may be going on with their client. If a therapist suggests to their client, for instance, that he may be giving away his power by overcontrolling those around him, this can be fleshed out right there in the office. The client may not resonate with this characterization and challenge the therapist to say more. Through sharing his experience of the client, rather than analyzing or interpreting the client's experience, the therapist might make it easier for the client to recognize what is going on for her in that moment.

When the therapist pays attention to his own body and shares what he feels, client and counselor explore together as a team, a partnership. For instance, "I'm aware of my own muscle tension growing in my back and neck as we talk, as if somehow I'm digging my own heels into the floor trying to push away." The therapist may ask the client to check out what he is experiencing to see if he feels something inside himself or about the therapist. Ultimately they may test out different ways of speaking to see if they each can either heighten or lessen the experience, providing them with data to interpret their experiment.

Clients sometimes engage in role-plays, which are more structured techniques for trying out something new. Susan is a client who had real difficulty asking her husband to meet her need for reassurance. Once Susan recognized how important it was to find different language to increase her impact, she rehearsed the exchange with her therapist. In rehearsing her assertions, she could feel herself growing stronger, more confident. This helped her to become more aware of her fears which grew simultaneously. The experiment allowed her to anticipate different outcomes and how she might feel and respond to them.

In a more challenging example, Tom had unfinished business with his deceased father. He was angry with his father, and it took him several months to realize this. Tom was rarely expressive of his anger, believing it was mean and disrespectful. He was willing to experiment with telling his father how he felt through imagining him in the room in order to experience how cathartic it was to be free of those feelings. He continuously checked with his therapist whether he seemed mean or disrespectful to ensure he wasn't violating any values he held. Expressing himself relieved a heavy burden that Tom had carried around for many years and gave him permission to be more honest with those in his everyday life.

An experience of reintegration *is ongoing, incorporating all those parts of ourselves that have been disavowed and helping us move from fragmented to whole.*

People are a complex web of many moving parts, the interaction between each of which forms a greater whole. There is our social self, wanting to fit in and be liked/accepted by others; our family self, where loving, commitment, and responsibility abound; and our work self, where creativity, perseverance, and industriousness are favored.

We can likely describe many facets of our personality, including our hopes, dreams, conflicts, frailties, attributes, and so on, that influence our humanity. Each of our many parts can be broken down into smaller components that connect us as human beings and make up our uniqueness as individuals.

As people, we tend to compartmentalize all the different parts because it suits us for the varied tasks and situations we encounter. The greater the compartmentalization, however, the more likely we are to become fragmented, like puzzle pieces that become disconnected. It is this experience that leads to many of the symptoms of discomfort in our lives.

This might be physical discomfort such as headaches, stomach problems, or back pain, or it might be emotional distress such as anxiety or depression. Discomfort can also be relational in terms of loneliness and alienation. Spiritual or existential discomfort includes a sense of being out of place in the world or questioning one's existence. The list is long of the possible areas that can be affected when we become fragmented, but the common thread is, what can be done about it?

In therapy we know that the whole is always greater than the sum of its parts. This means that it's the job of a therapist to help his or her client learn to integrate the self in a way that brings all the pieces together.

WHAT IS THE DIFFERENCE BETWEEN COUNSELING AND THERAPY?

While the terms *counseling* and *therapy* are frequently used interchangeably, there may be differences, depending on one's perspective. We can distinguish the two by examining the goals and methods of each. Counseling tends to emphasize a problem or a solution-oriented focus. Career counselors, for instance, help people develop needed skills or assist them in developing a plan for locating new employment or changing their existing job.

The term *counsel* means to offer advice or to advise a client regarding a particular dilemma. Some clients prefer a more pragmatic approach because it doesn't require the depth of contact that is more indicative of therapy. Counseling tends to emphasize shorter, more specific, and concrete objectives. The goals may be more measurable and the overall process may be less personal and more professional.

Therapy tends to emphasize an exploration of underlying issues and may be considered less pragmatic. Instead of focusing on a particular outcome, therapy pays closer attention to the process by which clients work toward their goals. For instance, if a woman comes into therapy because she is depressed, instead of simply providing strategies such as exercise, recreation, or socializing, therapy explores the nature of the unhappiness. What is keeping this woman from finding happiness so that the problem doesn't resurface at a later date?

A counseling psychologist is trained differently than a clinical psychologist, although confusingly the two professions may intermittently reference counseling and therapy. One particular difference in the training lies in the nature of assessment. Psychology training on the whole has the greatest concentration of diagnostic coursework, including objective, projective, intellectual, and academic instruments. Much more so than in social work, for instance, psychologists are trained to examine the causes of behavior, which is what allows them to administer evaluations.

Counseling psychology graduate courses include a cluster of employment-related courses such as the commonly used Myers-Briggs test. Counseling psychologists are more commonly found in academic institutions, where they help prepare college graduates for life after school. Clinical psychologists are more commonly found in mental health centers and in private practice, where people tend to seek out therapy.

Counseling is a term you will hear more often in school settings with children. A guidance counselor, school social worker, or school psychologist (master's degree) have "counseling sessions," which may take the form of crisis intervention or an assessment/referral process. Some school counselors meet with children on an ongoing basis in either individual or group settings. Group settings can help to build social skills, cope with a change, or work on other impediments to academic achievement.

School counselors also help mediate between teachers and parents when behavioral or academic issues arise. School counselors often have the unenviable job of serving as a school administrator in the disciplinarian role or dealing with outside agencies such as child protective services. Each counselor likely considers themselves an advocate for the children but also serves as a liaison for teachers who need help addressing institutional issues such as perceived inequity with their job.

School counselors tend to be the front line with peer relational issues in elementary and secondary education. The focus in high school in particular with juniors and seniors may be academic or vocational planning. The role of the school counselor often depends upon the interests and aptitudes of the counselor coupled with the needs of the school administrators. Some counselors, for instance, are well-trained clinicians who enjoy working in more depth with children, while others consider themselves experts in connecting families with community resources. Some counselors simply don't have the time to do what they are good at or enjoy depending upon the ratio of students in their schools and the frequency of crisis.

Overall, many professionals believe that counseling can encompass either definition and should not be limited or differentiated from therapy. It's advisable to check with the therapist you are considering working with to ask them about how they term their work and what differences if any they envision from the alternative term.

WHAT IS THE DIFFERENCE BETWEEN THERAPY AND COACHING?

Coaching, or life coaching as it is sometimes referred to, is growing in popularity. In our fast-paced, results-oriented society this modality of professional help is becoming more popular. Coaching is more convenient than therapy, in large part because it can be done by phone with greater convenience. Coaching also takes places via e-mail, providing greater flexibility in timing for those with busy schedules.

Coaching is a professional relationship, similar to that of a therapist, with confidentiality and other ethical constraints that are still universally agreed upon by various governing bodies such as the International Coaching Federation (ICF) http://www.coachfederation.org/index.cfm, International Society for Coaching Psychology (ISCS) http://www.isfcp.net/, and International Association of Coaching (IAC) http://www.certifiedcoach.org/, to name just a few.

Coaching helps clients identify and articulate specific goals and then assists clients in putting their very concrete objectives into place. Coaches first help you develop personal action plans designed to make behavioral changes, and then they help you develop strategies to maintain the changes you have made. Some coaches are generalists in that they work with a wide variety of needs, while others are more specialized. An example of a more specific coach is TeacherCoach (www.teachercoach.com).

Coaching is not reimbursed by insurance companies but can be made affordable. Oftentimes you determine how much you want to spend, and the coach will design a program accordingly. Other coaches give you different packages that fit your budget, which may even include group classes to reduce the cost.

Those who seem to benefit most from coaching are clients who are not looking to do in-depth work but instead want to make a specific, targeted change in their lives. This change can be in almost any area, including family, social, professional, spiritual, physical (health), financial, recreational, and so on. There is generally less vulnerability with coaching because there is less discussion of intimate topics. Those who are motivated and self-sufficient/independent tend to appreciate coaching because it seems to be a more balanced relationship with regard to power.

Coaching is not designed to help people with more significant concerns, such as those that compromise daily functioning. Trauma, significant emotional distress, entrenched relationship difficulties, and acute physiological turmoil are examples of matters better addressed in therapy. In-person sessions lend themselves better to helping clients achieve greater emotional vulnerability, which can be an important part of therapy, but it is not a crucial component in coaching.

The unique hybrid of coaching and therapy developed at TeacherCoach allows individuals to gain more immediate information and skills that aren't a replacement for therapy, but often a substitute or addendum. At TeacherCoach, people can opt for personal growth or professional development through coaching or classes. The same type of online resource will be available to anyone needing personal growth work at

TxHelper (www.txhelper.com) in 2015. The importance of immediate, convenient, and affordable help is the impetus for these sites, allowing people to benefit from self-help without the commitment or expense of therapy.

MY SENTRY . . . MY FRIEND . . . MY SELF (BY DEB R)

For a very long time I had been hiding behind what I referred to as "walls." This is a familiar representation in our group, and we have grown accustomed to and comfortable with this term. Those of us who feel imprisoned by these "walls" speak frequently and hopefully about chipping away and knocking them down. I also worked toward these goals to no avail. The harder I tried to destroy the walls, the stronger they became. I grew very frustrated and began to believe that my life would never be different and I would never feel joy again. I was being misled. By my own self.

Over the course of time I began to realize that the metaphor "walls" stood for an external and tangible force that I hid behind. In fact, there is no such structure around me. The force that protects and guards me comes from within. I began to understand that at some time during my life, probably when I was very young, I created a guardian "persona" or sentry to keep the evils of the world at bay. My sentry became very, very adept at preventing me from being hurt, thus I felt no pain. She prevented me from attempting challenges, thus I felt no disappointment. She eventually learned to prevent me from connecting with others, thus I began to feel nothing.

At first, following this ah-ha moment, I was actually very angry with this sentry side of myself. I plotted and planned ways to get rid of her, to destroy her. This, of course, was not very successful. I finally realized that this sentry was part of me, the person, and I would never destroy her because self-preservation is our strongest drive as humans. No wonder she fought long and hard to avoid being "knocked down," just as I would. Grudgingly, I began to have a sort of respect for her for the exceptional job she had done. She had taken over for me when I could no longer cope, and she had never, ever taken a break. She actually had more commitment and follow-through than I had ever given myself credit for. We began the slow process of calling a truce.

I began to understand what caused her creation in the first place and how her responsibilities had grown as my own life became more complicated. I also realized that she was getting weary. She had done a great job for a long time. She wanted to come home and rest. As I embraced her for the first time, I felt a love for her that I really didn't believe would ever be possible. I was proud of her for the fantastic job she had done for such a very long time. She worked so hard for me all those years, and yet she never once cried or complained. She kept things in control for me and took the brunt of all the bad things life throws at you and all the stress so that I could focus on the other things in my life. No wonder she became so tired.

I have called my sentry, and now my friend, home to rest. She is still resistant to give up her post. She is worried about whether or not I can handle being hurt or fearful or anxious. Like a mother guarding her young, she has a hard time letting go. I work every day to convince her that it is now time for me to care for her. I can only hope that as time moves on I can do as good a job for her as she has done for me. Every night before I go to sleep, I say my prayers to God and I tell my guardian, "Rest easy, my friend . . . a job well done."

Interesting Facts

- In 2012, an estimated 9.6 million adults aged eighteen or older in the United States had serious mental illness in the past year. This represented 4.1 percent of all U.S. adults.[6]
- Mental health problems lead to more than 150 million visits to physician offices, clinics, and hospital outpatient departments each year, making it one of the top three reasons why Americans seek medical treatment.[7]
- Countless studies show that while psychotherapy helps those living with depression and anxiety, drug therapy has become the most popular course of treatment over the past decade.[8]
- As depression diagnoses among the sixty-five-plus crowd become more commonplace—rising from 3.2 percent to 6.3 percent from 1992 to 2005, according to a nationally representative survey of Medicare enrollees—so, too, have medication-only treatments. Over that same period, the percentage of Medicare enrollees diagnosed with depression who were treated with antidepressants rose from 53.7 percent to

67.1 percent. The proportion of those who received psychotherapy, on the other hand, dropped from 26.1 percent to 14.8 percent (*Journal of the American Geriatrics Society*, 2011). Older adults aren't the only ones experiencing this trend. An analysis of two nationally representative surveys of U.S. households, for example, found that 75 percent of patients with depression were given antidepressants from 1998 to 2007, while the percentage of those who received psychotherapy dropped from about 53 percent to 43 percent over the same period (*Archives of General Psychiatry*, 2010).[9]

• The U.S. Surgeon General reports that 10 percent of children and adolescents in the United States suffer from serious emotional and mental disorders that cause significant functional impairment in their day-to-day lives at home, in school, and with peers.[10]

2

HOW DOES THERAPY WORK?

STAGES AND PHASES OF THERAPY

Therapy has three phases—assessment, intervention, and termination. These are not easily differentiated, because all three are ongoing, concurrent processes, intertwined to a large degree, and some might argue they're not different at all. Offering our experience of a person, for instance, to help them increase their own awareness may be evaluative in nature, but it's also a tactic on the part of the therapist to stimulate growth. If I suggest to a young male client that I notice how quickly we are speaking to each other and ask if he has noticed, together we are engaged in making meaning of my experience. I am sharing my perspective, which could be categorized as evaluative.

Assessment, in general terms, is the ongoing formulation of the person as they exist within their environment, how they seem versus what they present (congruence), and what they believe they need in contrast to what the therapist believes they need. This may also include the level of awareness the client has, the degree of integration or disintegration as it exists along different continuums, the level of distress the person is in, and their resiliency to tolerate the tension. Also assessed are the corresponding benefits and limitations of each approach taken by the client to find relief, the support system and the degree to which it is being utilized, and many more facets of the person's life.

At the same time the therapist is assessing their client, the client too is assessing the therapist. Therapists may not often encourage this direction of feedback, viewing it as a patient's transference (projecting feelings onto the therapist that originate elsewhere). However, encouraging a client to share what they liked and didn't like about the therapist/session sets the stage for ownership of the process, creating a continuous evaluation of what is taking place within the room. As opposed to the therapist guiding the course of therapy and the method by which the work is done, a partnership is formed which constructs therapy as a creative process of cooperative self-discovery. There are exceptions to this, however, such as psychoanalysis and some types of cognitive behavioral therapy, which are more structured and formatted. Encouraging clients to provide feedback about how they are assessing therapy isn't a threat to a therapist, but it may feel that way to some professionals. Therapists are human beings with the same insecurities and foibles as the rest of us. A therapist who isn't interested in balanced power or doesn't want to feel critiqued may overemphasize their role as expert, discouraging a healthy consideration of the process.

For clients who are overly passive, this can generate dependency on a therapist and discourage self-sufficiency. For those lacking in self-confidence, having a therapist provide answers as an expert can be deceptively attractive. Increasing our reliance on a therapist to the point where they make the decisions for us or provide constant "expert advice" gives us an easy out. If it doesn't go well, we have somebody to hold accountable, and if we are successful, we can't feel the full reward of accomplishment.

Intervention, the second phase of therapy, is the way in which the therapist positions themselves to aid in the goals of their client. A therapist actively intervenes when they stop listening and begin speaking, even if the utterance is an attempt to understand and convey empathy to a client. While this could simply be relating, early in the therapy process the remarks of the therapist may hold greater value, in particular if the client is looking for a prophetic phrase that could improve their life.

As will be discussed in more depth later, their theoretical orientation and other aspects of their training largely determine the way a therapist intervenes. Intervening can be as subtle as where the therapist chooses to sit in relation to the client or as direct as what homework assignments they suggest.

Assessing and intervening may occur simultaneously and interchangeably throughout the therapeutic process. Our current health-care model suggests that assessment is a one-time process, but a therapist is never done assessing their client, as people are always changing within their ever-evolving environment. Every time a therapist intervenes in some way, they are also attending to the impact of their involvement, which too can be considered assessment. An intervention is at times even aimed at both assessment and helping.

For instance, as a client is explaining the nature of his or her "problem" at their first session, a therapist may offer feedback such as, "It seems you have put great energy into figuring this out on your own but don't fully appreciate your effort." Here the therapist may be checking to see how the client accepts their affirmation, whether they are aware of their work, and if they are giving themselves full credit (versus focusing on the outcome only). This intervention is also aimed to provide support and let the client know that the therapist is on their side, recognizing their strengths.

Thus, we can differentiate assessment and intervention, but we appreciate that they often overlap and intertwine. The tasks of the intervention process are described, beginning with the process of building trust.

Rapport Building

Every client needs to feel a sense of safety, comfort, and trust in their therapist to be willing to divulge personal matters and look inward. The location of the building, the milieu of the office, the way the administrative staff handles clients' introductory calls, and how accommodating a therapist is for new appointments all influence a client's initial experience.

A therapist knows how important it is for a client to feel comfort, safety, and trust; however, they aren't always aware to what degree a client perceives these needs being met. A therapist may inquire how a client is feeling early in the session and even ask for feedback about the steps leading up to their first appointment. If you are asked how easy it was to get to the office or how the directions were, you know that the therapist is interested in his or her impact on you and not just what brings you to the office. This is a key component in forming trust.

If a therapist demonstrates a genuine eagerness to hear your reaction, rapport will be formed more easily. Your needs are specific, and the therapist's willingness to adapt his or her approach to meet these needs may put you at greater ease. This isn't to say that a therapist may alter his or her beliefs or style, but the pacing of the session, the degree of challenge, and the level of support can all vary greatly. Clients want to feel permission to test the waters by offering what is pleasing and displeasing to them as a way of assessing for themselves the degree of therapist receptivity and adaptability.

Perhaps the most prominent influence on a client's level of comfort is how well that client feels understood. If a therapist can demonstrate even a peripheral understanding of the various pieces to somebody's unique puzzle, clients may feel hopeful that therapy will be effective. Therapists know the importance of empathy (the act of putting yourself in somebody else's shoes and then communicating this experience), and they use a tool called *reflective listening* to make certain they are doing this well. Reflective listening is also called *mirroring*, because you are hearing back from the therapist what you are expressing, sometimes in different words. For example:

Client: "I don't know where to start. Should I just tell you about what's going on in my life right now or do you need some history?"

Therapist: "You're trying to decide where to begin . . . and looking for some direction from me, hoping I can guide you."

In this instance, the therapist recognized and appreciated the indecision and took the next step to support the client's choice of action.

Understanding can be provided at different levels of depth. In the above example, the therapist provided understanding at a very basic level. This is a safe way to communicate empathy, allowing the client to ease into his or her work. The therapist reflected the client's concern, putting the control back in his or her hands. Rapport is developing through both the understanding and the empowerment.

If the therapist were to have decided where he wanted the client to begin, it may have helped that client feel more directed, but it would also have established a different power differential. A more directive therapist may be appealing to some, but the clinician who encourages the client to assume their own power may be better appreciated.

In this next example, a more advanced form of empathy is demonstrated. Advanced empathy is used to build trust in a different way. It tells a client that the therapist is listening beyond the words he or she hears and into the deeper experience of the client. This experience may not always be known to the client, or the client may not be aware of it at that point in time.

> Client: "At this point I don't know what else to do. I've tried every-thing to get him to listen to me but nothing has worked."

> Therapist: "It sounds like you're feeling helpless. You're not very hopeful about seeing anything change."

This is an advanced form of empathy in which the therapist is reaching into what he or she has heard beyond the face value. This is a way of checking for deeper meaning beyond the immediate awareness of the client.

Rapport is created in different ways but is largely based on expecta-tions. Is the client expecting a wise old sage with a beard who ponders his words deeply as he inhales deeply into a pipe, or a maternal, motherly looking woman who seems touched by the client's circumstances? The picture we form of what we imagine therapy to be is oftentimes based on media depiction, stories, books, movies, and other venues, which don't often provide an accurate picture.

It is important to consider all the influences that have shaped our initial picture to gain an appreciation of what our expectations are. From these expectations we form standards by which we measure at least our initial experience in therapy. We want to have some idea of what would be helpful to us while being flexible enough to experience a new way of understanding ourselves which may be unfamiliar. As we explore our hopes and expectations, we will gain a better sense of how well the therapist we have chosen can accommodate us.

Discovery (What is causing these problems/symptoms?)

The search for answers is what therapy is most known for. If you watch any television program or movie, the therapist provides a framework for the client to understand the nature of his or her concerns. From the more analytical interpretation of problems, such as Barbra Streisand in *The Prince of Tides*, to the more compassionate and empowering approach of Robin Williams in *Good Will Hunting*, the search for answers is the thrust of therapy.

Clients often describe "symptoms" to their therapists, much the same way you would describe an illness to your physician. With a medical doctor (MD), a diagnosis is given with a prescriptive approach to treating the problem. You have little say in the treatment, and you measure success on the efficiency with which a solution is formed. With a doctor of philosophy (Ph.D.), or the more recent doctor of psychology (Psy.D.), the emphasis is on partnering with the client to reach a common goal.

The medical profession was built on a premise that a doctor's job is to aid the body in its own natural healing process. We have moved away from this in medicine and arguably in psychology. Instead of helping a person determine their own healing path, we have developed healing strategies we attempt to apply to each person to hasten the process. While this can seem initially successful, we must question whether it is actually healing or remedying.

Imagine how wonderful it would be if your medical doctor spent time with you exploring the causes of your ailment, inquiring into your nutrition, exercise regimen, stress level, hygiene, and other factors that may be at the root of your dis-ease. Instead, we have come to expect a quick fix that oftentimes includes medication. Perhaps this reflects the quickened pace of society or the impact of managed care, but it does not enhance accountability for our own health. It's a reactive approach that leaves little room for prevention and reduces long-term maintenance.

The paradoxical theory of change is not a widely held perspective among therapists but one that holds the utmost importance for appreciating the nature of discomfort and what is needed for long-term change. Simply put, nothing can be different until we appreciate why it already is. In a practical sense, we don't just get rid of anxiety until we know why it's there. Many cognitive behavioral approaches appeal to a client who believes his or her "symptoms" can be alleviated with techniques or strategies designed by the therapist. This is the quick-fix model that managed care and our own need for immediate gratification has moved us toward. The problem is that quick fixes can often be short-term in nature.

Consider the amusement park game (whack-a-mole) where moles pop out of different holes and the player punches them down with a soft mallet. Every time the moles get pushed into their hole, a new one pops up. This is similar to short-term therapy that promises immediate symptom relief. You may feel better in the short term, but it is possible that similar or related problems will pop up.

In gestalt therapy, the approach I take in my practice, you explore why a particular problem exists, knowing on some level it's directly related to who the person is and how that person lives. A client with chronic stomachaches, for instance, has discomfort located in this part of the body for a certain reason. The client could have headaches, back problems, or other physical ailments, so why their tummy? Before we help with relaxation training or other tension-relieving activities, we want to explore the message this body is sending. The body knows no way to communicate with us other than "symptoms," so we don't want to turn down the volume of these messages prematurely.

Ultimately, it's in the person's best interest to learn how to listen to what their bodies are telling them, so that discovery can be incorporated right into their own awareness, limiting the likelihood therapy will be necessary.

Experimentation

Once you have begun to gain insight about the nature of your concern, your options for action immediately expand. Take, for instance, a woman who comes to therapy with crippling anxiety. She works hard with her therapist to make sense of her panic, exploring both her external and internal stressors. She makes sense of her powerlessness experienced within her family and the resulting tension within her body.

The tension in her body is produced by trapped energy from not expressing her feelings and swallowing her anger. With the help of her therapist, she realizes that she is re-creating similar dynamics in her current relationships that existed as a child. With her husband, she would rather deal with the internal turmoil than she would an external conflict with him, so she avoids arguing at all costs. She blames herself for problems but ultimately cannot fool herself to believe her rationalization.

So, what is next? The issue at this point is that she knows intellectually that taking such a passive stance with her family is hurting her, and her body is letting her know through tension (experienced as anxiety). She fears making any changes for many reasons. This is the role she has assumed for many years, and it's familiar. She believes she can control the level of peace in the family by acting as a barometer. When it seems that others are on the precipice of a disagreement, she can insert herself into the dialogue with humor or another distraction. If she abandons this role, won't the family fall apart? She even fears rejection from others should she assert herself by expressing real thoughts and feelings. So, her resistance to change is strong.

The next step is to create an experiment. An experiment is a way of attempting something different, without feeling committed to a long-standing change. An experiment is a way of testing the waters, either by doing something different or by doing more of the same. This latter example would be used if the client wasn't convinced his or her action or inaction is creating a problem. So, for instance, in this example, if the woman did not believe her passivity impacted her anxiety, we might set up an experiment to help evaluate this potential connection. In the case above, however, we have established at a cognitive level that a connection does exist, but there is a healthy unwillingness to make a change— hence the experiment.

The best experiments are the ones you, the client, design. This way you can control the level of risk, the circumstance in which you are willing to engage, and other parameters that elevate the potential for safety and success.

Preparing for various outcomes is important for experimentation. I often tell clients that if we measure success by how others respond, we are setting ourselves up for disappointment. Of course, people are not always ready or interested in us changing our role/approach. It throws off the homeostasis we have created within our family system. Instead, we might view receptivity as an added bonus that is not to be expected. If this client were to assert herself with her sister (she selected the safest person to start with) and it resulted in a more honest and productive exchange, wonderful. But this ought not be the primary goal. Instead, we want to evaluate ourselves based on how we experienced ourselves with this new action.

Remember that the only certainty we have is that doing the same thing gets us more of the same response. Doing something different produces the unknown. The unknown will initially be something to fear and avoid but in time will become a source of curiosity which we seek eagerly. "When you hear the sound of the cannon, walk toward it."

So, this experiment designed by the client to assert herself with her sister has produced an unexpected reaction. While she initially felt fear (different from anxiety because fear is about doing something, whereas anxiety is generally about anticipating something that hasn't happened), she soon after felt powerful. As Carol Gilligan (a very early feminist psychologist) wrote about the process of finding your voice, when this happens, the energy that would have recycled back into the body (by not asserting the self) has been expelled in a way that leads to catharsis.[1]

For men, let me use a different example. If you have ever watched a boxing match or a baseball game, you will concur that more energy is expended by throwing a punch that is not landed or swinging at a pitch without making contact than is expended for a connection.

So, we evaluate this experiment on what it was like to be more genuine in self-expression. We appreciate both the unappealing outcomes as well as the appreciated ones. Most important in this experiment was the client's absence of anxiety. We don't know what future problems will occur, but it's safe to say there will be some. Every change we make has a ripple effect that produces some unexpected outcomes. We then have a choice to return to the way of old, doing what we had done for years, or to continue experimenting with something different. Sameness is familiar and oftentimes comfortable, but it also means not getting needs met, which is when our bodies start to rebel. We may listen to this rebellion by acting on our needs, or suffer the consequences. For some, this may mean medication to quell symptoms, or for others, it may mean illness, injury, or other types of incapacitation.

Assimilation

Once a client makes sense of what's going on for him or her and has added the experiential component that solidifies this understanding, that client can begin to put it all together. A man, for instance, who knows (cognitively) that his high anxiety is the product of all-or-nothing thinking plus the high expectations he holds for himself, and has solidified this insight with an experiment designed to heighten his anxiety (spend the week thinking everything has to be at one extreme or another), is ready for the next step.

This next step is called assimilation and may last for weeks or even months. It's like having the outline to a puzzle put together and starting to work on the inside. The picture begins to take shape as all the parts of the whole are coming together.

This stage of therapy should not be interpreted as, "I'm healed." Making sense of a selected issue or set of issues is exciting because it's usually the product of a lot of hard work. This is just one picture in a much larger collage that you are starting to make sense of. Insights do seem to come quicker at this point because you are mastering the process by which work is accomplished.

Long-Term Self-Discovery

While not every client enters into this phase of therapy, for those who aren't simply looking for symptom relief, it is likely that long-term self-discovery will be part of their work. When clients come into therapy, they don't often estimate how long they may remain in treatment, so it's not something you may know until you are engaged for a period of time exceeding three to six months. Very few clients announce their intention for very brief work, and most clients say they will be there as long as it takes. Now, this can be interpreted differently depending upon the nature of the client's work. Clients who find early symptom relief and resolve the presenting issue that brought them to therapy gratefully terminate their sessions with the option to return at any later point in time. For others, the work becomes an important part of their lives.

The trap of therapy, so to speak, is that the more work you do on yourself, the more work you find you want to do. Personal growth work can be intoxicating. When the sense of urgency has dissipated and you are creating successes through your experimentation, you may want to do this work at deeper levels. People operate similarly to an onion that can be peeled layer after layer. Those who learn to tolerate the sting in their eyes continue to explore themselves closer to the core.

Many of those who begin to enjoy this work, much like going to the gym or having a personal trainer, build therapy into their weekly routine like any other commitment. Some opt to join group therapy (discussed later), which is a more affordable and enjoyable way of doing self-discovery work.

Termination is the third and final phase of therapy. Even in long-term therapeutic relationships, an end point starts coming closer from the very beginning of therapy.

Therapy starts the moment the first phone call is made. When you extend yourself to a professional to ask for help, you are placing your trust in another person. At the start of therapy, this trust is not yet formed;

however, you are sharing very personal aspects of your life, both past and present, in order to help the therapist form a picture of your life.

The first several sessions are imbalanced, in that the client is working considerably harder due to all the risk taking and information sharing. The therapist often remains quieter, allowing the client to share what he or she is willing to divulge, occasionally asking questions for clarification. During this period, the therapist is searching for strengths and limitations of the client's approach, understanding his or her needs, and generally trying to figure out how to best help the client.

Toward the middle and end of the first session, the process goal formation (to be described in more detail later) occurs. Because the immediate objective tends to be the development of a plan of action, the client isn't necessarily going to "feel better" at the conclusion of the session. They may feel unburdened, however, from finally opening up to somebody while feeling hopeful from starting the process of therapy. The opportunity to ventilate the body of some tension that has been stored within can be quite cathartic.

First sessions may run longer than the traditional forty-five minutes, depending upon the therapist. Because this time seems to go by very quickly, it can help to prepare before going in, which will be addressed in chapter 8. For now, it's okay if you have so much to talk about that you feel "all over the map." The therapist may take notes during the session, but even if he or she doesn't, that therapist is well trained to remember the key points of what you outlined.

Even when you have certain goals visualized, those goals will likely change as therapy goes on. Therapy involves ongoing evaluation of your goals, because the more you learn about yourself, the clearer your direction becomes. It's like driving along a windy, mountainous road with frequent signs for falling rock. You rarely end up where you intended because of the unexpected obstacles. Goal setting in therapy is more like pointing to a spot on the map that moves, sometimes by degrees and sometimes by time zones.

Therapy can be a process of transitional change; incremental change; or, most frequently, transformational change. Transitional change may include surviving a divorce, grieving a loss, or even blending of a stepfamily. Incremental change is about taking small steps toward a very specific goal, such as those seeking "anger management." The most rewarding type of change is the last one, the kind that places greater emphasis on the journey than the destination.

So, what is it about this journey that makes it so important? Consider the following illustration to help this idea make sense:

John rushes home from work each day, frustrated by traffic and agitated by his fellow drivers. While at first he is eager to see his family, he arrives home grumpy and wanting to be alone. In this repeated pattern, John is determined to reach his desired goal, without attending to the process by which he is reaching it.

Throughout the therapy process, the therapist provides consistent feedback to help stretch your perspective. Since we typically view the world through a particular lens, we routinely act upon the same information in similar ways. Say, for instance, we perceive a coworker as bossy, always telling us what to do. Our reaction to this perceived bossiness is perhaps to get defensive and/or to avoid the person. It is safe to say that we would deal with like people in similar ways, not recognizing the role we play in this exchange.

Through therapy we might explore why our sensitivity to being "bossed around" is high, not recognizing where our reflexive response is coming from. Of course we can justify that "everybody" experiences this coworker in the same way, not having to look at where our reaction is stemming from. A therapist may help you pay attention to what is being brought up for you; say, for instance, a feeling of insecurity that is evoked through the perception of an authority figure abusing their power or a sense of helplessness that reminds you of something from your past or present.

During these sessions, your therapist will provide empathy, or a demonstration that he or she understands your feelings, allowing you to move past your fear of judgment into a more exploratory stance about who you are and how you came to be. As you feel better understood, your defenses may lower, opening you up to greater self-exploration. Not only does feeling understood allow someone to find validation, it helps them look beyond their protective mechanisms into their core self.

In your therapy, you will likely gain useful tools to help you negotiate your needs with greater success. These tools are too numerous to mention them all but may include assertiveness training, visual imagery, relaxation techniques, or breathing exercises. By expanding your repertoire of useful intrapersonal and interpersonal strategies, you may find more peace and harmony with the world.

Sometimes therapy is not about change but about accepting ourselves for who we are, flaws and all. In fact, identifying those aspects of ourselves we typically hide for fear they will lead to rejection from others are the very facets of our personhood that build intimacy with others.

Termination is an unpleasant word because it's associated with death, firing, and endings which stir up rejection and abandonment. In therapy, termination is the move toward independence. Everything accomplished in therapy is part of termination because it's building on strengths, skills, and possibilities. Although many leave therapy prematurely, those who have a planned and thoughtful ending will find it easier to return to therapy if needed, feel more accomplished about what they have gained, and start the next phase of life more clear about where they have come from.

Termination is a good-bye with a good friend that is likely to bring us sadness and hurt, which is why it's talked about from very early on and then consistently through the therapy process. If people wait until the end to talk about the ending, they may uncover issues that they didn't realize were there, elongating therapy and leading to disappointment.

White Flag

Exploring myself . . . deeply,
Stop being on the "surface" with myself and others,
I want to fill the void.
Overcome fears and anxieties.
Open doors that have been locked and forgotten.
I want to cry, laugh—I want to feel.
Be vulnerable . . . so I can let myself in.
How can I let others in—if I can't let myself in?
I feel separated from myself . . .
There is me, then there is "me."
I want to become whole. When that occurs . . . maybe I will not feel so empty inside.
I want to become positive and look forward—rather than be negative and look . . . no stare . . . at the past.
I want to love . . . not hate.
Feel success . . . not shame.
Be happy . . . not sad.
Burn every damn mask I wear!

Feel free!

I want to be light . . . not heavy or weighed down.

I want peace within myself.

Stop hiding from the pain.

Stop hiding from the world.

I want to wake up in the morning and not want to be so eager to sleep at night.

I want the battles to stop within myself.

This is my white flag . . . my surrender!

Catherine K

3

WHY DO PEOPLE GO TO THERAPY?

WHY IS IT HELPFUL?

According to the National Institute of Mental Health, nearly 27 percent of Americans aged eighteen and older (one in four adults) suffer from a diagnosable mental illness, an estimated fifty-seven million people. [1] Nearly 5 percent or almost three million children are reported by their parents as having serious emotional or behavioral problems. In addition, millions more Americans who may not meet criteria for a serious mental illness seek help dealing with issues seeming beyond their control, such as problems with a marriage or relationship, a family situation, loss of a job, the death of a loved one, unhappiness, stress, burnout, or substance abuse. Those losses and stresses of daily living can at times be significantly debilitating or can at least diminish our quality of life.

People generally seek therapy for two different but broad reasons. The first and most common reason is personal crisis. Our marriage or relationship may be in jeopardy, our children may be struggling, or we ourselves may be experiencing hardship that threatens our personhood. Crises range in severity from confusion to outright turmoil. When we face a crisis, it often means our usual coping mechanisms are not working as they once did, and/or our capacity to tolerate the distress has diminished.

A second reason for seeking therapy is an interest in personal growth. "I am content in my life but I want to be fulfilled." "I feel like I don't know who I am anymore, as if I have lost my identity." Sometimes those who begin therapy in crisis move toward this type of less urgent but equally important work. When people come to therapy for more self-discovery-designed work, the work looks different. Instead of concrete, specific goals that are measurable, the work takes on a more existential flavor. Questions about Who am I? What do I stand for? mean in-depth soul searching that has no clear beginning or end.

Life is full of challenges. We encounter roadblocks to happiness at every turn in the busy highway of life, and sometimes these hurdles seem too high or too frequent to navigate. We grow tired and sometimes we stumble. We may even fall and not have the strength to get back up.

Sometimes the emotional weight of these challenges can put a strain on your system, creating messages from the body we in this society refer to as "symptoms." These messages, or symptoms, can be back pain, stomachaches, headaches, fatigue, or a range of hundreds of sensation clusters.

Oftentimes we start out by ignoring these messages, either because we are "too busy" or hoping our situations will improve and our lives will get easier, but sometimes we seek out help to feel better. Others are more sensitized to bodily changes and react more quickly, even catastrophizing the irregularity as something major. In both instances, our distress manifests physically, leading us to address the matter with our primary care physician (PCP).

Some may check in with their PCP first, hoping to rule out physiological causes to these symptoms. We may receive medications or other suggestions for dealing with or eliminating the problem, but in relying solely on this approach, we may be missing important messages our bodies are sending us about more psychologically based needs.

This doesn't mean we are imagining or making up our ailment; in fact it's quite the contrary. Stress is like trapped energy in the body that creates havoc on our regulatory systems, leaving us with very real maladies. The question is on what level are we looking or willing to address these issues.

WHO SEEKS THERAPY?

Years ago somebody who "needed therapy" was assumed to be crazy and was believed to have some deep-seated psychological problems that made

Table 3.1.   Sample Symptom Checklist

Symptom	Possible Message from the Body	Unmet Need/ Conflict
Stomachache	Let go of fear	Security
Neck tension	Narrowed range of focus	Control
Unmotivated	Lack of quality fuel	Freedom
Worry	Detached from body	Security
Indifference	Not getting enough reward	Power
Agitation	Holding in tension	Independence
Back injury	Overburdened	Support
Dysphoria	Battery low	Fun/excitement
Mood swings	Be vigilant	Stability
Sleep trouble	Need catharsis	Resolution
Weight gain/loss	Insulate for safety and loneliness	Affiliation

him or her the center of attention, like wearing a big scarlet letter "C" for Crazy on their chest. If not pitied, he or she was ridiculed or shunned.

We imagined these individuals lying on the couch of a stereotypical psychiatrist who sits behind the couch, notepad in hand, searching for hidden meanings in their dreams. Our fantasies of what went on in these closed-door sessions were the stuff of movies:

> Psychiatrist: "So, you are dreaming about a vast desert, stretching for hundreds of miles with only a single cactus standing desolate in the center of this barren wasteland. And you say the cactus has the face of your mother-in-law, the body of your boss at work, and your dog's tail. Well, I think it's clear what's going on here . . . you are confused about sex!"

With the help of films and television shows such as *Dear John*, a self-help support group for middle-aged men and women; the ongoing neurosis of Woody Allen, who brought his therapy into every film; Frasier, a psychiatrist with his own radio talk show; and *Dog with a Blog*, a kids' show featuring a psychologist dad, we have begun to view therapy with curiosity and interest. With the help of the media, we have learned that it's the most ordinary people who seek therapy, because those who are genuinely crazy don't know enough to seek help or may not benefit much if they did.

Those who are willing to put time, money, and energy into their personal growth are also likely to value accountability. With the number of obligations and responsibilities each of us has, it is admirable for somebody to invest himself or herself in personal growth.

People come to therapy for many different reasons. Some are in acute distress, such as those experiencing intense anxiety or depression. Likely having waited until their discomfort grew so strong they are having difficulty functioning in their daily activities, therapy became a matter of urgency. These consumers of therapy initially look for relief from their distress and care less about how to attain it.

Others come into therapy not because they are in pain, but due to a desire for something greater. They are not satisfied with their lives and believe greater fulfillment is out there waiting to be found. It is this second group that tends to stay longer in therapy, because they are not looking for the "quick fix."

Interesting Facts

- More than 50 percent of adults and 70 percent of children and adolescents are not receiving any treatment for their mental illness. [2]
- Mental illness usually strikes individuals in the prime of their lives, often during adolescence and young adulthood. All ages are susceptible, but the young and the old are especially vulnerable. [3]
- Individuals living with serious mental illness face an increased risk of having chronic medical conditions. [4]
- Adults living with serious mental illness die on average twenty-five years earlier than other Americans, largely due to treatable medical conditions. [5]
- African Americans and Hispanic Americans used mental health services at about one-half the rate of whites in the past year and Asian Americans at about one-third the rate. [6]

COMMON ISSUES

Anxiety (Generalized Anxiety, Panic Attacks, and OCD)

Everyone feels anxious or stressed from time to time. Situations such as meeting tight deadlines, anticipating important social obligations, or driving in snow/heavy traffic often bring about worrisome feelings. Such mild anxiety may help make you alert and focused on facing threatening or challenging circumstances.

Anxiety disorders cause severe distress over a period of time and disrupt the lives of individuals suffering from them. The frequency and intensity of anxiety involved in these disorders may be debilitating. But fortunately, even severe anxiety is often dealt with effectively with therapy alone. There are several major types of anxiety disorders.

People with generalized anxiety disorder have recurring fears or worries about health, finances, or other daily life activities, often accompanied by a persistent sense of dread that something bad is just about to happen. The reason for the intense feelings of anxiety may be difficult to identify. But the fears and worries are very real and often keep individuals from concentrating on daily tasks.

Panic disorder involves sudden, intense, and unprovoked feelings of terror and dread. Those who suffer from this disorder generally develop strong fears about when and where their next panic attack will occur, and they often restrict their activities as a result. For those who are unsure what is happening, the experience can be made more frightening by the apparent similarities between a heart attack and a panic attack, sending many to the emergency room every year.

A related disorder involves phobias, or intense fears, about certain objects or situations. Specific phobias may involve things such as encountering certain animals or flying in airplanes, whereas social phobias involve the fear of social settings or public places.

Obsessive-compulsive disorder is characterized by persistent, uncontrollable, and unwanted feelings or thoughts (obsessions) and routines or rituals in which individuals try to prevent or rid themselves of these thoughts (compulsions). Examples of common compulsions include washing hands or cleaning house excessively for fear of germs, or checking over something repeatedly for errors.

Someone who suffers severe physical or emotional trauma, such as from a natural disaster or serious accident or crime, may experience post-traumatic stress disorder; returning combat veterans are often prone to this disorder. Reminders of the event seriously affect thoughts, feelings, and behavior patterns, sometimes months or even years after the traumatic experience.

Symptoms such as shortness of breath, racing heartbeat, trembling, and dizziness often accompany certain anxiety disorders such as panic and generalized anxiety disorders. Although they may begin at any time, anxiety disorders often surface in adolescence or early adulthood. There is some evidence of a genetic or family predisposition to certain anxiety disorders.

If left untreated, anxiety disorders can have severe consequences. For example, some who suffer from recurring panic attacks avoid at all costs putting themselves in a situation that they fear may trigger an attack. Such avoidance behavior may create problems by conflicting with job requirements, family obligations, or other basic activities of daily living.

Many who suffer from an untreated anxiety disorder are prone to other psychological disorders, such as depression, and they have a greater tendency to abuse alcohol and other drugs. Their relationships with family members, friends, and coworkers may become very strained. And their job performance may falter.

Most cases of anxiety disorder can be treated successfully by appropriately trained health and mental health-care professionals. Although the National Institute of Mental Health shows research that both "behavioral therapy" and "cognitive therapy" can be highly effective in treating anxiety disorders, other less well-known approaches can be just as, if not more, helpful.

Individual, family, and group psychotherapy (typically involving individuals who are not related to one another) are common approaches for treating anxiety disorders. While some seek relief through medication, it is suggested that a person meet with his or her therapist first before taking this step. Although antianxiety medicine may help us function more easily, the medicine may mask important information from the body.

Several principles help people in therapy to successfully reduce anxiety. Shifting the focus from outcome to process is one. If we take pressure off ourselves to achieve certain results, measuring success based on how we went about addressing certain tasks, we shift the control from external to internal.

If we move from overthinking to utilizing our bodies, anxiety will also diminish. Anxiety can be thought of as overreliance on our brains, helping us to anticipate problems of the future or ruminate about what has already taken place—with the goal of improving outcomes. If we spend more time paying attention to our bodies, our sensations in particular, we will locate our needs more easily and be able to take steps to meet them.

Anxiety can also be seen as trapped energy in the body. If we locate where the energy has been trapped, we can recognize how we have been holding back so that we may work toward being more assertive in our relatedness. Those who learn to address conflict can feel more internal peace as opposed to maintaining external peace.

Interesting Facts

- Anxiety affects forty million adults in the United States aged eighteen and older (18 percent of the U.S. population). [7]
- Anxiety disorders are highly treatable, yet only about one-third of those suffering receive treatment. [8]
- Anxiety disorders cost the United States more than $42 billion a year, almost one-third of the country's $148 billion total mental health bill. [9]
- More than $22.84 billion of those costs are associated with the repeated use of health-care services; people with anxiety disorders seek relief for symptoms that mimic physical illnesses. [10]
- People with an anxiety disorder are three to five times more likely to go to the doctor and six times more likely to be hospitalized for psychiatric disorders than those who do not suffer from anxiety disorders. [11]
- Only one out of four people with panic disorder receive treatment. [12]
- Approximately one out of seventy-five people may experience panic disorder. [13]

Depression

According to the National Institute of Mental Health, an estimated 18.8 million adult Americans suffer from depression during any one-year period. Many do not even recognize they have a condition that can be treated very effectively. Distinguishing clinical depression from feeling down, sad, or gloomy can be difficult. [14]

Everyone feels sad or "blue" on occasion. Most people grieve over upsetting life experiences such as a major illness, loss of a job, a death in the family, or a divorce. These feelings of grief tend to become less intense on their own as time passes.

Depression occurs when feelings of extreme sadness or despair last for at least two weeks or longer and when they interfere with activities of daily living such as working or even eating and sleeping. Depressed individuals tend to feel helpless and hopeless and blame themselves for having these feelings. Some may have thoughts of death or suicide. Those who are depressed may become overwhelmed and exhausted and stop participating in certain everyday activities altogether. They may withdraw from family and friends.

Changes in the body's chemistry may influence mood and thought processes, such as our menstrual cycle, illness/injury, adolescence, or long-term deprivation. Biological and genetic factors also contribute to some cases of depression, although we still aren't certain to what extent. In addition, depression may accompany chronic and serious illnesses such as heart disease or cancer. For many individuals, however, depression signals first and foremost that certain mental and emotional aspects of life are out of balance.

Significant transitions and major life stressors such as the death of a loved one or the loss of a job can bring about depression. Other more subtle factors that lead to a loss of identity or self-esteem may also contribute. The causes of depression are not always immediately apparent, so the disorder requires careful evaluation and diagnosis by a trained mental health-care professional.

Sometimes an individual has little or no control over the circumstances involved in depression. At other times, however, depression occurs when people are unable to see that they actually have choices and can bring about change in their lives. Feeling powerless and without hope are key components of depression, and if someone can be helped to feel more powerful and in charge of their future, improvement is likely.

Some stigma, or reluctance, is still associated with seeking help for emotional and mental problems, including depression. Unfortunately, feelings of depression often are viewed as a sign of weakness rather than as a signal that something is out of balance. The fact is that those with depression cannot simply "snap out of it" and feel better spontaneously.

Persons with depression who do not seek help suffer needlessly. Unexpressed feelings and concerns accompanied by a sense of isolation can worsen depression. The importance of obtaining quality professional health care cannot be overemphasized.

Psychotherapy offers people the opportunity to identify the factors that contribute to their depression and to deal effectively with the psychological, behavioral, interpersonal, and situational causes. Skilled therapists can work with depressed individuals to pinpoint the life problems that contribute to their depression, and to help them understand which aspects of those problems they may be able to solve or improve.

A trained therapist can help depressed patients identify options for the future and set realistic goals that enable these individuals to enhance their mental and emotional well-being. Therapists also help individuals identify how they have successfully dealt with similar feelings if they have been depressed in the past, which is often the case.

The work in therapy often includes the realization of hidden energy that has become trapped in the body, to the extent that a person becomes flat, even immobile. As someone loses their will to take action, needs become less likely met, while feelings of hopelessness intensify. Through therapy we borrow energy from the therapist to take important steps toward wellness. This may include personal care efforts, activities that bring pleasure, the development of meaningful relationships, the need to resolve issues from the past that embody us with regret, and a sense of purpose that comes from making contact with the world.

If a therapist has a full appreciation of the simple but powerful idea that therapy may be the one place a client doesn't feel alone, then healing will already begin. Remembering that the only thing worse than pain is to be in pain while feeling alone will help us put the relationship first. While not all therapists believe that a meaningful relationship is a high priority for therapy (some wanting to remain more detached and analytical), keep in mind that the approach should fit with your needs. If you require neutral and surgical-like intervening, then you may find a therapist who focuses on the past or your thinking/behavior more helpful.

Most people, however, find that a genuine relationship with someone who sincerely cares for them is important for their personal growth. If we know a therapist likes us as a person and is invested in our well-being, we may feel safe enough to address the sensitive issues that have helped to create our depression. Through a healing relationship, a therapist may also help us in the following ways:

- Identify negative or distorted thinking patterns that contribute to feelings of hopelessness and helplessness that accompany depression. For example, depressed individuals may tend to overgeneralize; that is, to think of circumstances in terms of "always" or "never." They may also take events personally. A trained and competent therapist can help nurture a more positive outlook on life.
- Explore other learned thoughts and behaviors that create problems and contribute to depression. For example, therapists can help depressed individuals understand and improve patterns of interacting with other people that contribute to their depression.
- Help people regain a sense of control and pleasure in life. Psychotherapy helps us see choices as well as gradually incorporate enjoyable, fulfilling activities back into our lives.

One episode of depression greatly increases the risk of another episode, so make sure that you work not only toward the relief of discomfort, but to also shore up your fortification so that future distress can be handled with a lower risk of serious decline. There is some evidence that ongoing psychotherapy may lessen the chance of future episodes or reduce their intensity, but we aren't going to stay in therapy just because we want to prevent another episode. The idea of therapy is to be able to function in a world that mimics the openness and support of therapy, so we work to create this type of environment in our lives.

Therapists help depressed individuals and their loved ones in other ways. The support and involvement of family and friends play a crucial role in helping someone who is depressed. Individuals in the "support system" can help by encouraging a depressed loved one to stick with therapy and to practice the coping techniques and problem-solving skills he or she is learning through psychotherapy. Loved ones can also avoid judgments, advice, and empty platitudes that serve no purpose.

Living with a depressed person can be very difficult and stressful for family members and friends. The pain of watching a loved one suffer from depression can bring about feelings of helplessness and loss. Family or marital therapy may be beneficial in bringing together all the individuals affected by depression and helping them learn effective ways of coping together. This type of psychotherapy can also provide a good opportunity for individuals who have never experienced depression themselves to learn more about it and to identify constructive ways of supporting a loved one who is suffering from depression.

Medications may be very helpful for reducing the symptoms of depression in some people, particularly for cases of moderate to severe depression. Some health-care providers treating depression may favor using a combination of psychotherapy and medications. Given the possible side effects, any use of medication requires close monitoring by the physician who prescribes the drugs and hopefully consultation between all the treating professionals.

Some depressed individuals may prefer psychotherapy to the use of medications, especially if their depression is not severe. By conducting a thorough assessment, a licensed and trained mental health professional can help make recommendations about an effective course of treatment for an individual's depression. Those therapists who are less prescriptive may emphasize a more phenomenological approach, emphasizing a less pragmatic focus. For these therapists an exploration of the subjective reality is what helps clients appreciate why and how they become stuck.

Depression can seriously impair our ability to function in everyday situations. But the prospects for recovery for depressed individuals who seek appropriate professional care are very good. By working with qualified and experienced therapists, those suffering from depression can help regain control of their lives.

Interesting Facts

- An estimated one in ten adults report symptoms of depression. Even more people deal with lower levels of sadness that interfere with daily living.[15]
- Approximately 20.9 million American adults, or about 9.5 percent of the U.S. population aged eighteen and older in a given year, have a mood disorder.[16]
- Major depressive disorder is the leading cause of disability in the United States for ages fifteen to forty-four.[17]

- Major depressive disorder affects approximately 14.8 million American adults, or about 6.7 percent of the U.S. population aged eighteen and older in a given year. [18]
- An estimated 5.8 percent of men and 9.5 percent of women worldwide will experience a depressive episode in any given year. [19]
- Depression often co-occurs with anxiety disorders and substance abuse. [20]
- Approximately six million American men suffer from depression. [21]
- Nearly twice as many American women as men are affected by depression. [22]

Addiction

Substance abuse is a serious health concern; depending upon the severity, it can even be life threatening. Certain drugs are just as dangerous to be on as to withdraw from, so all treatment to become sober must include medical monitoring, which may even be done on an inpatient basis.

Addiction treatment has become a specialized field within the broader heading of mental health. There are various approaches to treating drug and alcohol abuse/dependency and different levels of care. The most intensive level is known as detox or residential treatment, where the addicted person might spend weeks or months in a structured program with physicians, counselors, and other health-care professionals.

Partial hospitalization is an intermediary step for a patient who does not qualify for inpatient treatment but needs daily attention to work on their addiction. The next level down is called intensive outpatient (IOP). In IOP, clients may go two or three times a week for several hours, mostly in group therapy. Finally, there is traditional outpatient therapy, which is the focus of this book. Not all therapists work with addictions in their private practice, and some people need to look to social service agencies or hospital settings for help.

In outpatient therapy, the therapist and client work on several issues, including relapse prevention, intra- and interpersonal relationships, family matters, and other underlying issues that coincide with or produce the addictive behavior. Many therapists subscribe to the disease concept model, which requires its members to attend Alcoholics Anonymous (AA) or Narcotics Anonymous (NA) meetings on a regular basis. Even family members are encouraged to attend their own twelve-step meetings to address their role in the addiction.

This approach works well for some; however, like any approach, it has its limitations. Complaints about this model include an overemphasis on religion/spirituality, a rigidity of philosophy, a discomfort with group settings, and a wish to get more to the core of the dysfunction.

Several other theoretical models have overlapping methods of intervention, so selecting the right approach is crucial to long-term sobriety and recovery. Sobriety and recovery are differentiated because someone can be sober without having worked through the myriad of issues that contributed to their addiction.

In any model you select for your treatment provider, it is important to explore the way contact is made with self and others. Contact is the way in which individuals experience life and informs the way in which we seek to get needs met. A typical addicted person will use substances to diminish contact within, blocking out important sensations from the body that signal when needs or conflicts are present. Using alcohol or drugs reduces self-awareness, not allowing the person to act on the messages from their body, but instead turning down the volume on immediate distress.

Due to the ongoing physiological risk of toxicity from drug/alcohol withdrawal as well as the consumption of these harmful substances, it is often recommended that medical consultation accompany any type of therapy. Therapists are not always trained in assessing the health risk of recovering addicts, so a team of professionals, including a nutritionist, is often beneficial.

Sexual "addiction" is also in this genre because it's viewed as a compulsion with qualities similar to substance abuse. This category may include an overreliance on pornography, serial infidelity, or the use of prostitution. Predominantly men deal with this issue, often feeling intense shame that inhibits seeking help, until they are in a crisis. This issue is born out of a major challenge that human beings face to sustain intimacy over a long period of time, combined with a sense of inadequacy and inability to tolerate distress.

Oftentimes those who suffer from one of the different sexual disorders will seek help through SA (Sexaholics Anonymous). While it can be helpful to have a support system to hold one accountable, the risk is that individuals may not look deeply enough into the nature of their struggles.

This is not simply a behavioral disorder in need of greater accountability, but a matter of socioemotional maturation. In-depth individual therapy coupled with group therapy can be helpful.

Eating Disorders

In a society that places a high value on thinness, even with the growing trend toward obesity, a high percentage of people worry about their weight at least occasionally. Those with eating disorders take such concerns to extremes, developing abnormal eating habits that threaten their well-being and even their lives.

There are three major types of eating disorders. People with anorexia nervosa have a distorted body image that causes them to see themselves as overweight even when they're dangerously thin. Often refusing to eat, exercising compulsively, and developing unusual habits such as refusing to eat in front of others, they lose considerable weight and may even starve to death.

Individuals with bulimia eat excessive quantities of food in binges, then purge their bodies of the food. They may also attempt to lose weight through the use of laxatives, enemas or diuretics, vomiting, and/or excessive exercise. Often acting in secrecy, they feel disgusted and ashamed as they binge, yet relieved of tension and purged emotions once their stomachs are empty again. Like people with bulimia, those with binge-eating disorder experience frequent episodes of out-of-control eating. The difference is that binge eaters don't purge their bodies of excess calories.

It's important to prevent problematic behaviors from evolving into full-fledged eating disorders. For example, very strict dieting and weight loss usually precede anorexia and bulimia. Binge-eating disorder can begin with occasional bingeing. Whenever eating behaviors start having a destructive impact on someone's functioning or self-image, it's time to see a highly trained mental health professional, such as a licensed therapist experienced in treating eating disorders.

According to the National Institute of Mental Health, adolescent and young women account for 90 percent of cases.[23] But eating disorders aren't just a problem for the teenage women so often depicted in the media. Older women, men, and boys can also develop these disorders. And an increasing number of ethnic minorities are falling prey to these devastating illnesses.

People sometimes have eating disorders without their families or friends ever suspecting that they have a problem. Aware that their behavior is abnormal, those with eating disorders may withdraw from social contact, hide their behavior, and deny that their eating patterns are problematic. Making an accurate diagnosis requires the involvement of a licensed psychologist or other appropriate mental health expert.

Certain psychological factors predispose people to eating disorders. Families in which boundaries are skewed toward enmeshed or disengaged may play a role, especially when one or both parents are highly controlling, critical and emotionally numb, or erratic. Personality traits also may contribute to these disorders, such as rigidness, repressiveness, and low risk taking. Most people with eating disorders suffer from low self-esteem, feelings of helplessness, and intense dissatisfaction with the way they look.

Specific traits are linked to each of the disorders. Those with anorexia tend to be perfectionistic, for instance, whereas those with bulimia are often impulsive. Physical factors such as genetics also may play a role in the level of risk.

A wide range of situations can precipitate eating disorders in susceptible individuals. Family members or friends may repeatedly tease people about their bodies. Individuals may be participating in gymnastics or other sports that emphasize low weight or a certain body image. Negative emotions or traumas such as rape, abuse, or the death of a loved one can also trigger disorders. Even a happy event, such as giving birth, can lead to disorders because of the stressful impact of the event on an individual's new role and body image.

Once people start engaging in abnormal eating behaviors, the problem can perpetuate itself. Bingeing can set a vicious cycle in motion, as individuals purge to rid themselves of excess calories and psychic pain, then binge again to escape problems in their day-to-day lives. The rush that comes from purging can become intoxicating and therefore self-reinforcing.

Research indicates that eating disorders are one of the psychological problems least likely to be treated. But eating disorders often don't go away without professional help. Leaving them untreated can have serious consequences and even be life threatening. In fact, the National Institute of Mental Health estimates that one in ten anorexia cases ends in death from starvation, suicide, or medical complications like heart attacks or kidney failure. [24]

Eating disorders can devastate the body. Physical problems associated with eating disorders include anemia, palpitations, hair and bone loss, tooth decay, esophagitis, and the cessation of menstruation. Those with binge-eating disorder may develop high blood pressure, diabetes, and other problems associated with obesity.

Eating disorders are also associated with other mental disorders like depression. Researchers don't yet know whether eating disorders are symptoms of such problems or whether the problems develop because of the isolation, stigma, and physiological changes wrought by the eating disorders themselves. What is clear is that people with eating disorders suffer higher rates of other mental disorders—including depression, anxiety disorders, and substance abuse—than those without eating disorders.

Therapists play a vital role in the successful treatment of eating disorders and are integral members of the multidisciplinary team to provide patient care. As part of this treatment, a physician may be called on to rule out medical illnesses and determine that the patient is not in immediate physical danger. A nutritionist may be asked to help assess and improve nutritional intake, although this professional needs to be aware of current advances in their field and cognizant of the forces for sameness that can thwart healthy eating.

Once the therapist has identified important issues that need attention and has developed a plan with their client, he or she helps the patient replace destructive thoughts and behaviors with more constructive ones, particularly those involving realistic expectations of weight gain. The therapist and the client work together to focus on healthier ways of coping with distress while delving into the underlying issues that promote the pathology.

Simply changing thoughts and behaviors is insufficient. To ensure lasting improvement, patients and therapists must work together to explore the psychological issues underlying the eating disorder. Psychotherapy may need to focus on improving patients' personal relationships, developing boundaries (a sense of self), the ability to negotiate to get one's needs met, a comfort with conflict, a greater tolerance for distress, and outlets for tension that are more constructive. Some work to get beyond an event or situation that triggered the disorder in the first place may also be indicated. Group therapy also may be helpful to accomplish some of these objectives.

In many instances, people with eating disorders respond well in outpatient therapy. This disorder isn't helped quickly, however, oftentimes requiring long-term therapy that people come in and out of throughout their lifetime. Incorporating family or marital therapy into patient care may help prevent relapses by resolving interpersonal issues related to the eating disorder. Therapists can guide family members in understanding the patient's disorder and learning new techniques for coping with problems.

Support groups can also help to show the person they are not alone. Taking away the uniqueness of the disorder can be helpful but also dangerous if the client craves a stronger identity. Sending somebody to a support group where they compete for who is the thinnest can have an adverse impact on health.

Remember, the sooner treatment starts, the better. The longer abnormal eating patterns continue, the more deeply ingrained they become and the more difficult they are to treat. Eating disorders can severely impair our functioning and health. But the prospects for long-term recovery are good for most who seek help from appropriate professionals. Qualified therapists, such as licensed psychologists with experience in this area, can help those who suffer from eating disorders regain control of their eating behaviors and their lives.

Interesting Facts

- Approximately 35 percent of those with binge-eating disorder are male.[25]
- An estimated 5 to 15 percent of those with anorexia and bulimia are male.[26]
- Eighty-two percent of respondents believe that eating disorders are a physical or mental illness and should be treated as such, with just 12 percent believing they are related to vanity.[27]
- Eighty-five percent of the respondents believe that eating disorders deserve coverage by insurance companies just like any other illness.[28]
- Eighty-six percent favor schools providing information about eating disorders to students and parents.[29]

- Eighty percent believe conducting more research on the causes and most effective treatments would reduce or prevent eating disorders.[30]
- Seventy percent believe encouraging the media and advertisers to use more average-size people in their advertising campaigns would reduce or prevent eating disorders.[31]

Stress

"People are disturbed not by things, but by their perception of things."
—Epictetus

Stress is the by-product of a natural tension state that allows our systems to prepare for fight or flight. An optimal level of stress allows for greater functioning. Too little stress and we may be overly passive, and with too much stress we find ourselves losing it on the next person to cross our path. Sometimes we explode, which looks like conflicts with others, and sometimes we implode, which is where anxiety and depression come in.

No single definition fits everybody, because stress is a highly personalized phenomenon and can vary widely even in identical situations for different reasons (so what I talk about may not fit each person exactly). Here are some physiological indicators of stress that are fairly universal:

- Shallow and increased respiration leading to a lack of oxygenated blood
- Adrenaline secretion
- Heart rate and blood pressure soaring to increase the flow of blood to the brain to improve decision making
- Blood sugar rising to furnish more fuel for energy as the result of the breakdown of glycogen, fat, and protein stores (resulting in fatigue)
- Blood is shunted away from the gut, where it is not immediately needed for digestion, to the large muscles of the arms and legs to provide more strength in combat or greater speed in getting away from a scene of potential peril (heightened muscle tension)
- Faster clotting to prevent blood loss from lacerations or internal hemorrhage

All these physiological responses are potentially useful in the short term; however, repeated occurrences can alter the regulatory systems in the body. When this happens, our body sends us signals (symptoms) that indicate we need to take action. If we ignore these messages, the intensity increases until disease or injury occurs. This doesn't include the psychosocial consequences of not attending to our bodies.

Many of these effects are due to increased sympathetic nervous system activity and an outpouring of adrenaline, cortisol, and other stress-related hormones. Certain types of chronic and more insidious stress due to loneliness, poverty, bereavement, depression, and frustration due to discrimination are associated with impaired immune system resistance to viral-linked disorders ranging from the common cold and herpes to AIDS and cancer. Stress can have effects on other hormones, brain neurotransmitters, additional small chemical messengers elsewhere, prostaglandins, as well as crucial enzyme systems, and metabolic activities that are still unknown. Research in these areas may help to explain how stress can contribute to depression and anxiety and its diverse effects on the gastrointestinal tract, skin, and other organs.

Causes of Stress

Stress comes from at least three places:

1. The difference between our expectations and our actual experience
2. Unmet needs or needs that are in jeopardy/threatened
3. Feeling unprepared for or concerned about something we anticipate

Coping with Stress

How we cope with stress is a large determinant in whether we generate more stress or reduce our stress level. For instance, if we take actions that don't meet our particular need, we now feel the void of what was originally affecting us plus the additional guilt/upset about our behavior (e.g., if we eat when we are stressed, we may feel angry or ashamed). Our ability to change course toward a more productive outlet depends largely on our awareness of what we are doing.

Common but unhealthy coping strategies are often the reason people seek therapy, as opposed to stress itself. This means that medium to high levels of stress may diminish a person's ability to cope, but the unproductive response to stress will leave him feeling desperate enough to seek out professional help. Alcohol, shopping, eating, smoking, and sex are just a few ways that people try to reduce their stress level.

Whether we opt for a healthy or unhealthy outlet for stress is the result of our early life experiences (watching our caregivers); the type of stress (acute, meaning short term, or chronic, meaning ongoing); our internal/external resources; and our willingness to take action.

Areas of Stress

- Occupational (e.g., lack of autonomy, direction, satisfaction)
- Family (e.g., injury, illness, finances, grief)
- Interpersonal (e.g., conflict, lack of intimacy, loneliness)
- Intrapersonal (e.g., shame, guilt, remorse)
- Existential (e.g., What am I doing with my life?)

Ten Keys to Long-Term Stress Reduction

- Process versus outcome (path as opposed to destination)
- Greater balance in relationships (giving versus receiving)
- Improved expression/negotiation of needs
- Transforming expectations into wants
- Developing effective outlets for catharsis
- Implementing a healthy nutrition and exercise regimen
- Finding humor where you can
- Greater integration of self by acceptance of inequities
- Seeking meaningfulness to put life in perspective
- Living in the here and now

Interesting Facts

- The majority of illnesses people deal with are a direct result of lifestyle issues, such as diet, exercise, and stress.[32]
- Most people spend several times more hours engaged in work than play. We expend much energy at work and then spend our free time recuperating and not doing pleasurable activities.[33]
- Most people—80 percent according to Deloitte's Shift Index survey—are dissatisfied with their jobs.[34]

Other Issues

People attend therapy for many other issues, some serious and some more about adjusting to life's challenges. The more serious issues, such as schizophrenia and bipolar and personality disorders, require a clinician who is specially trained and experienced, such as a psychologist. Obsessive compulsive disorder (OCD) and post-traumatic stress disorder (PTSD) are good examples of debilitating problems that can resurface throughout a lifetime if the issue isn't dealt with comprehensively.

Non-life-altering but significant issues such as grief, phobias, sexual problems, and other adjustment disorders don't necessarily require a therapist who specializes, although it's often helpful to work with somebody who feels comfortable and confident with your concerns. Finding a therapist who feels like a good fit and demonstrates competence in the work you want to do will likely guide your decision to select that person.

WHO SHOULD ATTEND THE SESSION?

This is a question many first-time clients consider for their first session. The answer is determined by these three factors: Firstly, consider how comfortable you are going alone. If you are scared and would be at greater ease having companionship, then you could always have a friend or family member travel with you to the office and sit in the waiting room. If you are terribly anxious, they might even join you in the session.

Secondly, does the reason you are seeking therapy have anything to do with relationships, in particular with a spouse or significant other? Many wives will initiate therapy because of unhappiness in their marriage but want to check out the therapist first before bringing their husband. This may be okay, but remember that as soon as rapport begins, there may be some uneasiness for the partner. The partner may wonder what was said about them and feel immediately defensive. Some therapists may deal with this by offering the partner a session of their own, while other clinicians will insist the couple start out together.

Thirdly, is having somebody with you going to impede or buttress your work? If having a third person in the session may inhibit your disclosure, then you may consider coming alone. If you believe a third person can help shed light on your situation and support you in being more open, then you might have them with you for at least the first session.

DO ALL THERAPISTS SEE FAMILIES/COUPLES?

Not all therapists work with families or couples. In fact, couples and family therapy is as much a specialty or concentration area as is substance abuse or eating disorders work. The major difference between individual and family/couples therapy is the perspective of the therapist. A systems perspective is one in which a therapist is well aware of how an individual relates to others and their community. Systems therapists make their diagnostic impressions largely on the interpersonal functioning of the various subsystems within the family unit.

If you are working with an individual therapist and believe you may eventually want to include other family members in your therapy, you have a number of options. You can ask your existing therapist what their comfort level is with bringing additional people to the session. You may also want to ask the same question of those you are intending to bring, because they may feel awkward coming into your therapy. The relationship has already been established and an alliance has already begun around your needs. Navigating the assimilation of a new person(s) can be tricky and requires a lot of ongoing talking about each person's experience.

The least complicated way to deal with bringing somebody new into therapy is finding another therapist who can see you and your spouse or family. This is common practice because it keeps boundaries clear. If you want the two therapists to speak with each other, then you sign a release of information, and they can talk about whatever you designate as essential. Your individual therapist can often recommend somebody they know of who does family/couples therapy so you don't have to start from scratch in the search process. This is a particularly helpful way of getting a referral, because the therapist knows you and likely has insight into whom you would work well with.

THERAPY CLIENT REFLECTION: "JOURNEY OF FEELINGS" (BY DEB R)

I am a very sensitive person. I just truly realized this about myself. I have probably known it for a very long time but never admitted it. I prefer to be called compassionate. This denotes more sensitivity for others than for myself. To have compassion for others seems to describe me as less selfish about my own feelings, and, while I am very sensitive to the feelings of others, I tend to neglect my own. The ability to recognize and act on my feelings is a luxury that I have long denied myself. This denial did not start out as some type of self-sacrificing martyrdom but as a way to protect myself. My feelings get hurt very easily, and I found that by withdrawing and avoiding intimacy with others, I gained a certain control over the circumstances by which I would get hurt and thus avoided the pain that came with it.

My sensitive nature does indeed extend to others around me. I am acutely aware of the feelings of others. This, for me, is a double-edged sword. I can be very compassionate to others, and this is helpful in health care and I believe makes me a better professional. I have also learned to control my feelings, however, in these circumstances because I can become too involved and take "my work home with me." My ability to feel for others also gives me the ability to hurt back or "sting" when my boundaries have been crossed. From these experiences I have also learned to withdraw, sometimes emotionally and even physically. This withdrawal keeps me from feeling pain and hurting others but leaves me with many unresolved issues, thus increasing my feelings of isolation.

My sensitivity has also caused me to become very reactive to criticism. I hate to be criticized in any way, constructive or otherwise. To me, this is a personal attack, and I become very, very defensive. When I was younger, I took any form of criticism as an attack on me as a person. I did not differentiate between something I may have been doing and who I was. I desperately wanted to be accepted and liked, particularly in school, and any unkind comment immediately became a sign that I was "different" and not accepted. To counter the pain I felt over this, I adopted a demeanor that kept people at bay. I might have been seen as a snob or maybe a loner. Others thought that perhaps I had a different group of friends outside of school that related to my horses and riding activities. Unfortunately, I adopted the same persona with them, and so the cycle started. I have never really felt accepted by any particular group in my life, and this has been very isolating. My father encouraged this "get-them-before-they-get-you" and "never-let-them-see-you-sweat" ideology, and my mother was full of helpful suggestions and activity ideas to cultivate these "friends" in the groups that I so desperately wanted to belong. Neither of these methods taught me how to deal with my feelings or helped me to accept myself for who I was. I can only assume that their methods were the ones they themselves used and had no other ways to teach. I don't believe their methods worked well for them either.

I now find myself at a "crossroads." I can either walk the path well traveled and one I am most familiar with, or take the other direction. By taking the other road, I will have to learn to navigate an entirely different way, and I am unsure how to go about this. I can either blunder through on my own or ask those that I meet on the way for help. I will open myself up for making mistakes on my journey and maybe even being made fun of, but I could possibly meet some very remarkable people along the way. I guess, in the end analysis, I have already chosen my road.

II

Selecting a Therapist

4

SELECTING THE RIGHT THERAPIST—FOR YOU

Selecting a therapist can be difficult. We often rely on our insurance companies to tell us which providers are "on the list" or look through an online listing for providers in our area. We should not feel compelled, however, to work only with those clinicians who are part of the managed care panels for our insurance. For those who can afford it, paying for a therapist privately can help protect your privacy and give you more control over the number of sessions.

Many avenues to locating a therapist allow us to gain information about the therapist and their practice, long before making the call. Online referral sources include:

- American Psychological Association (www.locator.apa.org)
- Good Therapy (www.goodtherapy.org)
- HelpPro (www.helppro.com)
- Network Therapy (www.networktherapy.com)
- Psychology Today (www.psychologytoday.com)
- Therapist Locator (www.therapistlocator.net)
- Therapist.com (www.therapist.com)
- Therapy Tribe (www.therapytribe.com)

These sites will provide a broad range of information about the practitioner, sometimes including videos, narratives, and checklists of issues addressed. What these sites don't give you is a personal sense of each therapist. So use these sites to narrow down your search and select a few people you would like to hear from. The following section will offer you questions to pose during your initial conversations and ideas to consider when speaking with them.

INTERVIEWING THERAPISTS: TEN QUESTIONS TO ASK

1. How long have you been in practice?
2. What is your theoretical orientation?
3. How do you see change take place?
4. How directive are you?
5. Have you worked with _____ before?
6. What are your views on medication?
7. How frequently do you typically schedule appointments?
8. Is there a fee for missed or canceled sessions?
9. Do you work with my insurance?
10. How easy are you to get a hold of?

1. How long have you been in practice?

There are benefits to working with a therapist who has been practicing for a shorter period of time. First of all, more novice therapists will likely have great enthusiasm for their work; they are eager to please and to prove their worth. Younger or less-experienced therapists often charge less money and may be more flexible with regard to scheduling and/or payment options. Younger therapists also tend to present less as an "expert," which could be a potential turnoff for a client.

A younger therapist may also be familiar with the latest research because of the recency of their graduation.

As in many other professions, the longer you "practice," the more practiced you become. Although each individual has a unique situation, very similar underlying themes come up repeatedly with clients. An experienced therapist knows what to look for and has "experimented" with different approaches to achieve a desired outcome. More experienced therapists may be less inclined to personalize anger or upset that a client may inadvertently direct toward them.

Experience helps a therapist to be more certain of his or her orientation/philosophy of change, which is the most important variable. Feeling confident but not rigid in a theoretical orientation is more common with experienced clinicians.

2. What is your theoretical orientation?

Chapter 11 is devoted to this topic, so we will not go into depth here. Suffice it to say that before deciding on a therapist to work with, ensure they have a firm commitment to at least one philosophy that drives their work.

When considering what a therapist's orientation is, imagine what it would be like to work with someone employing this philosophy. Try to sense how well it fits with your own belief system or how well you think you might respond. Keep in mind that the most common or recognizable approaches may not be the most effective for you. Simple and common-sense approaches may be appealing, but they may also lack depth.

3. How do you see change take place?

Change was described earlier as an ongoing process that oftentimes creates distress. How a therapist views change can tell you a lot about the way that therapist helps people cope with this unyielding process. Asking this question may yield valuable information about the way the therapist operates along many continuums, including existential versus practical, nurturing versus challenging, empowering versus authoritarian, or directive versus less directive.

The therapist's role in the change process is also important. Some may see themselves peripherally involved with change, while others believe they are the instruments of change. Listen to how a therapist talks about their role once they have described the change process to see how you feel about their explanation.

4. How directive are you?

The degree to which a therapist is directive dictates how much he or she leads the session versus how much you lead it. A very directive therapist is likely to offer more feedback, give advice or suggestions, and tell you of his or her experience of you. A directive therapist may challenge you more and provoke more conflict. Clients who feel less motivation, are lost, or need a higher degree of accountability may be tempted to gravitate toward this approach.

Be careful of your agenda, however, in selecting a therapist toward this end of the continuum, especially if you have the fantasy that the therapist will fix you. Regardless of how directive a therapist is, the onus of responsibility for doing the work is squarely on your shoulders.

A less-directive therapist does not mean that he or she is passive or less skilled. It may mean that the therapist empowers his or her clients by evoking responses in you that lead to your own insight and self-direction. This type of clinician believes that providing the right conditions in therapy, such as unconditional positive regard and empathy, is sufficient to allow you to be helped.

5. Have you worked with _____ before?

A therapist may be very experienced as a general practitioner, but that doesn't necessarily mean he or she is ready or willing to work with your particular issue. A therapist in practice for thirty years, for instance, who has seen thousands of young women in therapy, may be averse to treating an eating disorder because of his or her own life experience.

Few therapists "specialize" in a particular issue, so be careful of using this language. Specific conditions need to be met before one can say they specialize, although they may still be competent to help with your particular issue. If a therapist has worked with your particular issue, you can ask how much of that work occupies their practice (what percentage) and how well the therapist enjoys addressing that issue.

6. What are your views on medication?

Therapists are not medical doctors (with a few exceptions), nor are they qualified to answer questions about whether or not a client ought to be taking medication. With that said, it is commonplace for a therapist to recommend that a client seek an evaluation from a psychiatrist (a medical doctor trained in psychotropic medication). Because therapists can have extensive experience working with clients who take medication, they may also be good sources of information for clients on the topic of medication.

It is helpful to know where your therapist stands on medication, because it could be a factor relevant to your experience. Some therapists are quick to recommend that a client seek an evaluation for medication before therapy has even been given a chance to help. At the other end of the spectrum are those therapists who have strong biases against medication and may believe that it is never indicated. A balanced view is represented by a therapist who doesn't rush to judgment and knows that the client is in the best position to know whether medication is needed.

7. How frequently do you typically schedule appointments?

Traditionally, therapists meet with their clients at least one time per week for the foreseeable future of therapy or until the client has met most or all of his or her treatment goals. Weekly appointments allow for sustained momentum where work can be easily continued from week to week. Any lesser frequency can make it difficult to build a relationship and/or work on established goals, depending upon the seriousness of the presenting issues. Some therapists have very busy schedules and attempt to meet with clients twice a month. This is an option to consider only if you believe your objectives will not require more in-depth work.

8. Is there a fee for missed or canceled sessions?

Almost every therapist has a policy for clients who miss or cancel a session within a certain time period, such as twenty-four or forty-eight hours before the scheduled appointment. It is helpful for a client to know about this policy up front because it indicates how the therapist operates. The most typical scenarios are (1) a fixed fee for a missed session or (2) responsibility for the full session fee (co-pay and contracted rate with the insurance company).

While it may seem inflexible or uncaring to have your therapist charge you for missed appointments, it prevents the therapist from building resentment, which can interfere with the therapeutic relationship. It also helps to hold a client accountable when he or she doesn't feel like attending a session, which often occurs when difficult issues are being tackled or there has been significant emotional drain.

9. Do you work with my insurance?

This will be addressed in greater detail in part III of this book, but it is important to know, if you are unable to pay for therapy privately. Not all therapists are contracted with your insurance carrier and may not be considered "in-network." If you don't have an out-of-network option with your insurance, then you might not be reimbursed for services. If you didn't get a list from your insurance company of participating clinicians, then you might ask this question early in your phone call.

Ask the therapist who gets authorizations and who tracks when sessions are used up. You never want to learn that your insurance benefits expired and now you are responsible for paying for the sessions that weren't covered by insurance.

10. How easy are you to get a hold of?

It might seem like a difficult or obvious question to ask, but whether or not your clinician is reachable can really make a difference. Many therapists see clients throughout their entire day, leaving little time for returning phone calls promptly. It is usual for a therapist to call clients back at the end of the day (or in the evening) unless they have a cancellation or other break earlier, so knowing the therapist's usual practice is helpful. This way, if your therapist waits several hours to return phone calls, you will not be anxiously waiting for the return call.

Asking this question also sends a message to the therapist that you are expecting they have a certain level of accountability. While therapists are not crisis counselors, immediately available to help you through emergency situations, they ought to be responsive within a reasonable time frame. Knowing this up front can help clients avoid potentially upsetting disappointments.

INTERVIEWING THERAPISTS: TEN QUESTIONS TO CONSIDER AFTER THE FIRST CALL OR IN-PERSON MEETING

1. Does the therapist seem genuinely interested or distracted?
2. How well do I feel listened to and understood?

3. Has he or she given me any useful feedback?
4. Do I feel a little hopeful that I can successfully address my concerns with the therapist?
5. As I look around the therapist's office, do I get the feeling that I could be comfortable spending some time here?
6. Where on the continuum of clinically objective/detached does he or she seem to be?
7. Is working with a therapist of the same/different gender/age/ethnicity going to matter?
8. Am I ready to make this kind of time/energy/monetary commitment?
9. What might be the challenges of working with this particular clinician?
10. Will I be willing to assert myself with this therapist if or when needed?

1. Does the therapist seem genuinely interested or distracted?

The first phone call may be a window into your experience of the therapist. Did the therapist seem rushed on the phone? Were they interested in hearing a synopsis of your situation so that they could determine if they were competent to work with you? Did you feel a sense of warmth or at minimum interest in your distress?

Oftentimes therapists are rushing to return calls quickly during their day, so there may be some urgency to hurry through the call, or in some situations you may speak primarily with a receptionist. If you aren't able to get a full sense of the therapist but feel interested in learning more, have a first session where you can better determine in person how they seem to you.

Therapists should not be answering calls during the session, and the majority do not take notes unless they are asked to perform some evaluative type of service. If we pay attention to how the therapist is paying attention, we can assess their level of engagement. If you find they seem distracted or not interested, let them know. There isn't a better determination of a therapist's value than how they respond to direct feedback.

2. How well do I feel listened to and understood?

Your very first conversation with a clinician gives you an idea of what to expect. While you aren't likely sharing deep or highly specific information on the phone, the clinician will likely ask for a vague description of why you are calling and what expectations you have. This is done to ensure that your issue is within the scope of competency for the therapist and whether he or she has confidence in helping you.

It is not uncommon, for instance, for a therapist to turn down a client who is struggling with a sexual problem, if that therapist believes this is outside their scope of practice. The therapist must not only convey a sincere appreciation for how you are feeling but also a sense that they are knowledgeable about the issue. One indicator of this may be if the therapist is able to tell you other ways your issue may impact you. If you hang up the phone saying to yourself, "They get it," then you are off to a good start.

Imagine you are a female in her mid-thirties calling because you have been experiencing panic attacks. During the conversation, the therapist recognizes how scary it is to have what can feel like a heart attack without warning. The therapist even goes beyond this by identifying that the harder you try to keep the panic contained, often the worse it gets. This helps you to appreciate that the therapist has worked with people suffering with panic and knows how out of control someone can feel, especially when their attempts to stop it don't help.

3. Has he or she given me any useful feedback?

More so in person than by phone, therapists will offer some type of feedback to assess your level of insight, receptivity, and willingness to look at yourself from another perspective. This can vary widely depending upon the style and theoretical orientation of the therapist, some of whom will spend a lot of time listening to gather all the information they can early in therapy.

Other therapists are less interested in data and more attuned to what the impact is from your situation. Contextual factors become less important than the way you both protect yourself and open yourself up to growth that is occurring. For this reason, therapists may not offer feedback on the immediate dilemma, looking for patterns and themes which may emerge around the circumstances bringing you to therapy.

In both cases where therapists are more pragmatic and insight focused, feedback may be offered about what you are going through. Without this feedback you may feel as if you are simply telling your story without any input, leaving you uncertain how therapy is going to be helpful.

Ask yourself at the conclusion of the first few sessions what you have heard from the therapist that sounds similar to or different from talking with friends and family. There ought to be a distinguishable difference in the quality of the feedback you are receiving. If you haven't heard anything that impacts you, it's okay to ask them for feedback. How does what I'm presenting seem to you? What are you learning about me after I have shared all this information?

4. Do I feel a little hopeful that I can successfully address my concerns with the therapist?

This is a gut check for therapy, mixed with a more logical appraisal of the therapy. On a practical level, does the therapist seem intelligent? Does he or she seem to balance listening and speaking so it doesn't become too one-sided? Is this approach to working with me something that makes sense or at least seems unique to how I have been dealing with it? Keep in mind that therapists spend years in training that covers areas such as human behavior, personality, pathology, theory, and much more. The therapist should sound knowledgeable.

You can't answer this question through your intellect alone, because hopefulness is also experienced through the body. So pay attention to your energy and whether it rises through excitement (the hope of finding somebody who can help) or gets bottled up into anxiety (I don't know if he or she is right for me). Along with your gut, ask yourself whether this person feels comforting, challenging, accepting (but not complacent), and interested.

Putting together our brain and body will help us to make the most informed decision. If you don't get a sense of them on either a thinking or a feeling level, it's important you express this concern to the therapist to gain their input. Circumstances that don't involve the therapist themselves could be impacting you.

5. As I look around the therapist's office, do I get the feeling that I could be comfortable spending some time here?

Once you've had your initial appointment, you will be able to assess the therapist in a number of different ways. How comfortable was the waiting area and how conducive was it to privacy and peacefulness? How helpful was the receptionist with the complicated process of getting you authorized through the insurance and explaining to you the bundle of paperwork you filled out? Did the therapist explain his or her policy on confidentiality and make clear the limits to your privacy? What is their policy on canceling appointments, and does it sound reasonable?

Once inside the office, how comfortable do you feel? Are you seated on a couch or a chair that faces the therapist, or are there obstacles between you, such as a desk? Is there free space that helps you feel more exposed? Any objects or furniture may serve as barriers that interfere with contact, even though they may feel like they are keeping you protected.

What kind of decorations hang on the wall? Is the clinician licensed, with diplomas hanging on the wall, keeping in mind the sometimes thin line between expert and narcissist? We don't want our therapist to feel arrogant, as this will help us toward subservience and powerlessness.

6. Where on the continuum of clinically objective/detached does he or she seem to be?

Perhaps the most noticeable characteristic that impacts a first impression is the therapist's level of involvement. Where on the continuum is a matter of personal preference, based on factors that tell us something about ourselves. We may be looking for somebody who is warm and nurturing or more clinically objective, based on our level of trust, how much we are logic/reason driven, and what issues we are bringing to work on.

A clinician who seems concerned about you as a person may be appealing because you feel cared for. The pitfall of too much caring is a loss of objectivity that clouds a therapist's judgment. On the other end of the continuum is a clinician who seems extremely professional, so much so that you aren't able to make an emotional connection with him or her.

Thus, a middle ground between caring and clear boundaries may be the ideal.

7. Is working with a therapist of the same/different gender/age/ethnicity going to matter?

An initial consideration for new clients is the preferred gender of the therapist, which is going to vary from our initial consideration of therapy to our ongoing experience. This means you may have a strong preference when making phone calls, such as "I only want a female therapist." If you feel strongly about this, then go with your instinct.

But also remember that our instinct may lead us toward safety, which isn't in the direction of beneficial work. Leaning into our discomfort, whether it's to work on issues of same-sex relatedness ("I never seem to get along with other women") or opposite gender relations ("I am really struggling with my husband, so a male therapist may yield a helpful perspective"), will lead us toward a greater understanding of ourselves. This learning is done experientially, which means that our brain plays a less significant role, at least initially. Making meaning of where our discomfort comes from is a complex process requiring an experienced professional partner who can help us determine what part of ourselves to attend to and when.

Female clients oftentimes choose female therapists, suspecting they will feel better understood. Males may select male therapists, especially when the issues are of a sexual nature, fearing the embarrassment of talking with a woman. Women may steer away from females, fearing them to be judgmental, or away from males because they will minimize feelings. These concerns are largely based on our life experience, so awareness of our biases can help.

Gender can also be important when considering therapy for children and adolescents. Parents will assume their teen daughter prefers a female therapist, and in many cases this is the case. It's worth checking with your teen, however, because they may surprise you with their choice. If body image and/or eating disorders are part of their work, a quick conversation with the therapist by phone (male or female) may help parents and teens alike ease their discomfort. While the navigation of gender differences may be an unnecessary obstacle for the traumatized or frightened teen, others will find the opposite gender a fresh perspective. In particular for female teens, who are dealing with competition from peers, a male may help deemphasize self-consciousness.

With children, parents may feel safer with a female therapist. Males who work with young children are less common but are certainly plentiful. Young boys who are lacking a consistent male role model may find a male therapist appealing.

The issue of ethnicity has factors similar to yet different from those of gender. Similar cultural or ethnic backgrounds may yield greater appreciation for client experiences, such as the high expectations for males in Japanese families. We must remember, however, that extreme variability exists within all ethnicities, so sharing the same background isn't necessary. A qualified therapist will explore differences in moral, religious, and ethnic backgrounds as well as sexual orientation, becoming a student to learn their client.

Many therapists will seek advanced training in areas such as work with gay, lesbian, and transgendered clients, so asking what their training has been will be helpful.

8. Am I ready to make this kind of time/energy/monetary commitment?

The decision to partake in therapy is a major one because it involves a considerable amount of time, energy, and money. Setting aside at least an hour a week is not easy, particularly when someone feels pressured to accomplish all the obligations already present in his or her life.

For those who are serious about improving their lives, be prepared to work outside the forty-five-minute therapy "hour." If your only work (a term used to describe the therapy process) is done in the office, you will find your progress slow. The learning you extrapolate from inside the session to your life will be where growth occurs. Whether this is in the form of risk taking around assertiveness, trying to be more "present" to reduce anxiety, or joining a recreational activity to improve happiness, the work extends well beyond therapy.

Energy is another factor to consider in deciding to commit to therapy. It can be draining to open up about suppressed feelings, especially if you find yourself highly guarded. Working through pain will involve strong resistance, which is the force for sameness pressuring you to keep it safe. With this in mind, consider what type of energy reserve you have and what you will do to keep your energy stores up during the early phase of therapy, where exhaustion can be highest.

The effort needed to make important changes can extend well beyond the session itself, which also can be challenging for someone who feels drained or low on motivation. Whether you are using insurance, making a co-payment, or paying privately for therapy, the cost can add up over time. Consider that a simple weekly $20 co-payment over the course of a year comes out to about $1,000 annually. It is for these reasons that you have to prepare yourself for this endeavor to remove as many barriers as possible.

9. What might be the challenges of working with this particular clinician?

Every therapist, no matter how helpful, is going to inherently bring certain qualities or conditions that can serve as perceived barriers to therapy. It can be as simple as an inflexible schedule that forces you to come during inopportune times or as complicated as talking about private aspects of your sex life with an opposite-gender therapist. Try to anticipate what challenges will exist so that you are not caught entirely off guard.

This might even be a question to pose to the prospective therapist: "What do you imagine the barriers will be to our working together?" or "What issues can you envision arising that might be challenging for us to work through?" If you have your own ideas, present them early and often.

A helpful therapist will welcome feedback you provide about the obstacles to therapy, helping you to feel as though your concerns are normal and worthwhile. Remember that you are the consumer and you have a right to voice your experiences, even if it means confronting the therapist. This can be uncomfortable if you view him or her as an "expert" that is rigid and beyond reproach.

10. Will I be willing to assert myself with this therapist if or when needed?

There will come a point, or many points if you remain in therapy long enough, when you will challenge your therapist. This ought not be viewed as defiance, arrogance, or a disregard for help, but instead as a natural response to the therapeutic process. You are your own expert and you have beliefs, opinions, instincts, and so on that may be opposite to the therapist's.

The important question to ask yourself is, What will you do when this time comes? Considering what your immediate response to such situations usually is can help let you know if this person is right for you. If you shy away from conflict, will this therapist help draw out your strength? If you tend to get combative, will the therapist be firm but nonreactive to your force? You might even experiment with this during the initial phone call or the first session. Test-drive your assertiveness early and see what the response is. If you are really bold, you can bring it to the therapist's attention and let him or her know what you are doing—this is sure to lead to a lively conversation that will give you helpful data.

KEY INGREDIENTS FOR THERAPISTS

While each client is going to find certain characteristics of a therapist helpful, other, less clear components will be important to consider. The following list is more complicated than may be useful, but for those interested in a more in-depth appreciation of therapists, it's something to consider.

1. **Use of Self:** Is the therapist aware of, open to, and interested in talking about their own experience of themselves with you? Are they willing to share their experience of you in a way that enhances rather than detracts from your work?
2. **Balanced Perspective:** Does the therapist concentrate on one aspect of you, such as your behavior or thoughts, as opposed to seeing all of you and how all the parts work together?
3. **Embodiment:** Does the therapist help you pay attention to sensations within your body to help you make meaning out of "symptoms?" Some therapists will be very present in the room, helping you bring issues to life to fully understand them.
4. **Self-Awareness:** How well does the therapist have a sense of how you feel about them, envision them, relate to them, etc.? We want and need a therapist who recognizes their own issues and what is being sparked inside the therapy session and who can distinguish their own "stuff" from ours.

5. **Limitations:** Does the therapist have a sense of where they are not serving their client well, may lack information or experience, or are stuck in a way that helps to stagnate therapy? Therapists need to know when they are not the best person to guide your work.

6. **Diversity:** Does the therapist appreciate and value difference, in particular with regard to ethnic, gender, racial, and sexual orientation, and other variances? Contact is made only through the exploration of uniqueness, as opposed to making everybody the same.

7. **Competence:** Has the therapist worked with and been trained in the matter(s) of importance to you? Are they willing to bolster their own knowledge base if they are uncertain or would benefit from continuing education?

8. **Hope:** Does the therapist believe they can be helpful in instilling a sense of hope that you will feel better? Do you end your dialogue with a sense of optimism that life will improve as a result of your work in therapy?

9. **Challenge:** Is your therapist willing to push you when you feel stuck, without having it feel like force? Helpful therapy involves some amount of leaning into our discomfort, which means having a therapist who isn't avoidant of sensitive issues or pain.

10. **Availability:** A therapist who fits all the above descriptors but can only meet with you once a month when you need something more regular can be an impediment. Are they willing to e-mail you occasionally between sessions and respond to phone calls in a timely manner?

5

THEORETICAL ORIENTATION

A theoretical orientation is a philosophy or a paradigm that one uses to guide their approach to therapy. Not all clinicians subscribe to particular orientations; in fact, most call themselves "eclectic" or "integrated," meaning they pull from numerous approaches. In this chapter we consider four of the main orientations; however, hundreds exist today. Nearly all of the orientations and approaches therapists use today have developed from one of the four main paradigms outlined in this chapter.

Consider the contents of this chapter with curiosity as opposed to striving for full comprehension. The goal is not to have you become an expert on the various philosophies and theories, but instead to gain a better sense of what resonates within you as most stimulating and appealing.

There are many ways to achieve an outcome; however, the method can vary greatly. How we ultimately achieve our goals can have as much to do with feeing successful as the outcome itself. Therapists have widely differing beliefs about how a client is best helped and what the clinician's role is in this process. In order to make a determination about the most effective help, understand something of the vehicle by which you are taking this important journey.

Since people seek out therapy because they want something to be different, we begin by asking how that difference comes to be. How the therapist views change, and what role he or she plays in facilitating this change, tells you the foundation of their philosophy. Change may be the elimination of uncomfortable "symptoms" such as tension, apprehension, and panic (anxiety); or lethargy, apathy, and dysphoria (depression). It may be the improvement of relationships through assertiveness training, development of trust, or creation of intimacy. Or change may be the attainment of greater joy/happiness in one's life through resolving trauma, reducing anger, or finding greater meaning in an area such as a career.

Theoretical orientation can also be referred to as the philosophy by which a therapist operates. Orientations differ significantly, depending upon several variables including the focus on past, present, or future; attention to mind, body, or behavior; how directive the therapist intends to be; and the continuum of insight to the strategy they employ. The role of the therapist, the nature of the intervention, and how one conceptualizes pathology (deviation from the norm or, in this case, health) are other dimensions that separate philosophies.

Understanding your therapist's orientation will help you understand what to expect from him or her and the process of therapy itself. You will also work together as a more effective team if you are each working from similar premises.

Below are summaries of some of the more common orientations. These are only a few of the hundreds of approaches/philosophies that exist. They have been selected because they are more established theories, seemingly separating some of the major camps of therapy. They also happen to be some of the oldest approaches, with familiar founders' names that include Sigmund Freud (psychoanalytic), Fritz Perls (gestalt), Carl Rogers (client-centered), and Aaron Beck (cognitive).

Consider the bias of this author as a purist, subscribing to gestalt theory and therapy. Recognizing the value of other approaches is important, but having the adaptability and creativity to borrow from other schools of thought is a key ingredient to successful therapy. Even within the four theories and their founders mentioned above, not one of them is practiced in the precise way the theory was first conceptualized. Many key pioneers have reformatted these approaches over the years; their names may not be mentioned, but their contributions are profound.

GESTALT

Gestalt therapy has two main functions. The first is to help people resolve unfinished business from the past and the second is to appreciate how the past impacts us in the present. The trauma, for instance, of being mistreated as a child has strong implications for both the lack of peace in the past and how we relate in our current lives. In addition to understanding the influences of this early event, we want to come to terms and find some level of acceptance so that we can move forward with our lives.

Gestalt therapy is about reaching our potential as human beings, doing so by bringing together all of our "parts" into a collective whole. We all have inherent greatness within our reach, but fragmentation (the parts of ourselves becoming more separate) occurs, leaving us feeling scattered. We tend to overemphasize certain parts, such as our thinking, which can lead to anxiety and depression. By overrelying on our brains, we lose sight of our bodies, which is where our needs reside. We begin to treat the messages from our bodies as "symptoms," resorting to "treatments" that only address the outermost edge of the issue.

The way we recognize our potential is by integrating our parts, removing obstacles (sometimes this is unfinished business), and recognizing our resistance, a naturally occurring struggle between sameness and change. This may include resolving fears of intimacy and facing distractions such as alcohol, food, gambling, or sex.

Gestalt therapy is based on the paradoxical theory of change—in order to make something different, you must fully understand what it already is. So, for instance, if you are experiencing anxiety, then before we introduce relaxation techniques to reduce the worry, we explore it to understand why it's occurring.

This philosophy is far from the quick fix that many seek when they want to eliminate discomfort. A gestalt therapist does not want to patch someone up only to see that person in six months with new problems. If getting your needs met were a simple process, each of you would have done so long before the signals from your body became so loud.

Contact is a central theme in gestalt work, describing the way in which we experience ourselves, others, and the world. Through contact we make meaning of what's taking place inside us, between us, and in our environment. Contact means having defined boundaries of who we are so that we can relate more fully, a prerequisite for intimacy between human beings.

When we take another person in fully, we also realize new aspects of ourselves. A husband who gets closer to his wife may become more aware of his fear of abandonment, only realized because of his growing intimacy. Contact is resisted for this very reason, the discomfort that often accompanies feeling vulnerable.

People ultimately realize through gestalt therapy that vulnerability is actually a misnomer, as we become stronger and more resilient through our availability to contact. Vulnerability is more about physical exposure, such as a ground troop invading a territory without air cover. In humans, being available to contact means being in touch with what we are feeling as well as the person we are relating with, willing to let them into our world.

We tend to resist this process, fearing exposure, humiliation, rejection, and shame as consequences of letting go. If we relinquish our protective mechanisms, we risk feeling out of control and susceptible to the attack of others. In actuality, what happens is that others feel closer to us because of our willingness to let them in, rewarding us often by returning the favor.

The body is strongly emphasized in gestalt therapy. Opposed to some other models, gestalt helps us become aware of those parts of ourselves which we have detached from, disavowed, or otherwise shut down. James Kepner analogized this to having a room in one's house which isn't frequented or even acknowledged to exist, yet is known to be there. It's common for people in Western culture to lose contact with their bodies. [1]

Whether we have been traumatized in some way growing up, have a poor body image, or simply overemphasize our thinking, our bodies tend to become trivialized or even objectified. A client once said, "I'm not sure why *it's* doing that," in reference to his body where he experienced chest constriction. In our society we tend toward symptomatology, which further alienates our body. If we pathologize (label with illness) this constriction as potential disease as opposed to a message from the body, we cannot make meaning of what is happening. Instead we treat only what is visible to us, like the tip of the iceberg sticking up out of the water.

Gestalt focuses on a person's health, their potential, their inherent goodness. Instead of disease, a gestaltist would say dis-ease, meaning one is experiencing distress that leads to physical health problems. Therefore, a primary objective of gestalt work is to improve our capacity for distress.

With a higher threshold for discomfort or distress, we have improved health and a greater range of choices to get our needs met.

It's sometimes difficult for clients to trust the theory behind gestalt therapy because it's less well known and not advocated for by physicians or managed care. Consider the client suffering with "irrational thoughts," as we call them in this society, such as fear of flying. She knows that the plane she gets on isn't *the one* that is going to crash, yet she fears it as if it's a certainty. This client believes strongly the problem is in her head and therefore her thinking needs to be "treated" with medication or cognitive restructuring. Getting in touch with her body may be received skeptically when the problem is clearly in her head.

Here is an example of potential dialogue between a gestalt therapist and a client:

Client: "I'm feeling so low on energy, I just can't seem to get myself moving."

Therapist: "Share what it's like to feel so stuck. See if you can describe the forces that want you to move and the ones holding you still."

Client: "I want to move because I have so much I have to do, but I'm holding still because none of the things I have to do I really want to do."

Therapist: "Perhaps the forces keeping you stuck are actually helping you realize how obligated you feel toward life, which interfere with what you really want to be doing."

COGNITIVE BEHAVIORAL

This approach may be the most well known to the general public. It is widely researched with the support of the managed care industry due to its reputation as a time-limited, easily monitored method of client care. In an age when insurance companies want—or require—requests for ongoing service or treatment plans to include measurable and observable goals and objectives, this approach is especially popular, as its strategies are easily framed in these terms. Most therapists, regardless of their treatment approach, describe goals in behavioral terms when requesting additional sessions from insurance companies and use forms such as treatment request forms (TRFs) or ongoing treatment requests (OTRs).

Cognitive behavioral therapy, often referred to simply as "CBT," approaches client care with the underlying assumption that our thoughts, feelings, and behaviors are inextricably linked. Consider the following plausible scenario:

While driving on a busy freeway, you are suddenly cut off by an unfamiliar vehicle while approaching your exit. You may think to yourself, "Didn't that jerk see my signal?!" This thought might be accompanied by feelings of frustration or anger and may prompt you to lay on your car's horn, engage in a colorful hand gesture, or even tailgate the offending vehicle.

Now consider the following additional piece of data: The exit you were about to take leads directly to an area hospital, and the car that cut you off is carrying a pregnant woman in distress. How does this impact the ways you interpret and react to the event of being cut off? Instead of believing yourself to be slighted, you may wonder whether the woman is safe, and feel concern for the family's welfare. With these internal experiences in mind, you may be less likely to respond with anger than you were before.

As seen above, the way in which we interpret events in our environments has direct implications for how we feel about and respond to those events. By exploring the bidirectional connections among thoughts, feelings, and behaviors, CBT aims to address clients through two major aspects of their personhood: thinking and doing. The theory behind a cognitive approach, for example, suggests that we each have an internal monologue that is consistently in motion—much like music on your computer or headset set to repeat indefinitely. By helping people to notice and evaluate the tracks on their personal playlists (sometimes called "hot thoughts" or "automatic thoughts"), a cognitive therapist's goal is to coach clients to recognize and exchange those unhelpful thoughts with ones that are more flexible, constructive, and personally effective. As clients gain mastery of this skill, they may discover new ways of responding to the environment, thereby engaging in behaviors that are more in line with their individual goals and values.

In addition to exploring the inner world of the client through his or her thoughts and the underlying beliefs that promote those thoughts, CBT therapists are trained in strategies to actively promote target behaviors while exploring their cognitive underpinnings. While less common in the professional marketplace today, strictly behavioral therapists focus on the form and function of those behaviors the client reports as unwanted. Imagine the parent of a boy who frequently engages in attention-seeking behaviors at home and at school, to the detriment of his academic and social functioning. A behavioral therapist might observe the child with the express purpose of identifying how "attention-seeking" looks; when these actions tend to appear; and how peers, caregivers, and teachers respond to the behavior. Armed with the results of this targeted detective work, the behavioral therapist is then able to develop a behavior plan with specific recommendations for how to respond to the child's behavior moving forward.

There are many ways to foster behavioral change, which at their core are based on the principles of reinforcement and punishment. In the case of positive reinforcement, the parent of the child above might provide an incentive such as a hug or a high-five when her son gains attention in a more appropriate way. On the other hand, she may apply an aversive stimulus or remove privileges to discourage inappropriate behavior such as physical discipline; these two responses are often called "positive" and "negative" punishment, respectively, within the context of therapy, as they aim not to promote the desired behavior per se but rather to decrease the frequency of the unwanted behavior.

In general, reinforcement tends to be a more effective means of shaping target behaviors, as the process provides the child with the specific message "You just did what I want you to do." Punishment serves as a less effective means of instilling intrinsic self-control, as it not only fails to let the boy know what he should be doing, but also requires constant feedback in order to reduce the frequency of unwanted behaviors, which may leave him feeling resentful or afraid of his caregivers.

Taken together, CBT aims to promote behavior change by addressing both the internal and external experiences of the client. CBT is at its core a present-focused treatment approach, with no immediate focus on the long-term origins of behavior. On the surface, CBT presents as a practical approach for those who are interested in reaching short-term, problem-focused objectives. There is considerable research on the efficacy of this orientation with those suffering from depression and anxiety as well as children with behavioral problems, making this a preferred approach for those who are more scientific and solution focused.

Here is a potential example of dialogue between a cognitive behavioral therapist and a client:

Client: "I'm feeling so low on energy, I just can't seem to get myself moving."

Therapist: "It's definitely hard to get started on anything when you're not feeling your best. What are some of the things you have to do?"

Client: "Well, my wife wants me to clean out the garage, and I'm falling behind at work and have to get some reports done, and my kid wants me to build her a tree house. It's just so much, and I'm feeling overwhelmed."

Therapist: "I would feel that way too! I wonder what it would be like to break one of those bigger tasks down into smaller pieces, and then start chipping away bit by bit. Not only will your work start to get done, but you might feel accomplished as you check things off your list and actually get back some energy."

PSYCHODYNAMIC (OBJECT RELATIONS, PSYCHOANALYTIC, SELF PSYCHOLOGY)

Psychodynamic refers to a cluster of orientations that examine the intrapsychic experience of the client, largely influenced by early childhood relationships and experiences. Sigmund Freud was a pioneer in the field, the originator of psychoanalysis, from which these other theories have sprung; however, many along the way have shaped more contemporary approaches still under this same heading.

The many different kinds of psychodynamic therapy include self psychology, ego psychology, object relations, and psychoanalysis. Each of these orientations is different in the way it conceptualizes and treats patients. A common thread among all the different subtypes is an emphasis on understanding the unconscious motives, conflicts, and drives of the patient. All of these perspectives seek to understand the patient's coping mechanisms as a way of identifying less-healthy adaptation within relationships.

The healing and change process in long-term psychodynamic therapy usually involves at least two years of sessions because of the complex goals of changing an aspect of one's identity or personality or integrating key developmental learning missed while the client was stuck at an earlier stage of emotional development.

The role of the therapist in traditional psychoanalysis is different than in other orientations, because the therapist or "analyst" is in more of an expert role. The therapist is something of a tabula rasa, or blank slate, onto which the patient projects thoughts, feelings, and fantasies—referred to as transference. This event is significant because it allows the patient and therapist to understand early-life experiences and current intra- and interpersonal dilemmas.

This orientation is best suited for individuals who are interested in understanding how they came to be. There may be less empathy and encouragement through this approach; instead, the focus is on insight and discovery. For people with deep-seated phobias, neuroses, and complex childhoods needing exploration, psychodynamic theory can prove valuable.

Here is a potential example of dialogue between a psychodynamic therapist and a client:

Client: "I'm feeling so low on energy, I just can't seem to get myself moving."

Therapist: "When in your life have you felt this way before? Go back to your earliest memories of feeling stuck."

Client: "I used to feel very scared as a child, so I didn't take many risks. Sometimes I felt so scared I couldn't even move."

Therapist: "Consider what was happening with you when you were feeling so scared as a child."

CLIENT-CENTERED (ROGERIAN)

Carl Rogers was one of the most famous therapists of all time. He was an extraordinary practitioner who could help someone who was simply in his presence. His warmth and compassion made him a unique therapist who has significantly shaped the way we look at human potential. He pioneered the move away from traditional psychoanalysis and developed client-centered psychotherapy, which recognizes that each client has within himself or herself vast resources for self-understanding, for altering his or her self-concept, attitudes, and self-directed behavior, and that these resources can be tapped by providing a definable climate of facilitative attitudes.

It is a nondirective approach to therapy, "directive" meaning any therapist behavior that deliberately steers the client in some way. Directive behaviors include asking questions, offering treatments, and making interpretations and diagnoses. Virtually all forms of therapy practiced in the United States are directive. Instead, Carl Rogers believed that certain conditions are necessary in therapy to help a person, such as empathy, unconditional positive regard, being nonjudgmental (acceptance), and others.

A nondirective approach is very appealing to many clients because they get to keep control over the content and pace of the therapy. The therapist isn't evaluating the client in any way or trying to figure out the client. Clients who work hard, have good insight, and appreciate being in control may benefit from this model.

People who are extremely motivated, insightful, and disciplined will thrive with Rogerian therapy. A greater sense of accomplishment is likely with this approach because as the client, you feel responsible for your gains, unlike other, directive approaches that teach or guide clients toward success.

Client-centered therapists tend to emphasize the relationship, helping you feel like a partner is working with you to navigate life's challenges. A partner who never judges and listens more intently than friends, parents, and spouses do allows you to build your energies and utilize your internal resources to take action.

Here is a potential example of dialogue between a Rogerian therapist and a client:

Client: "I'm feeling so low on energy, I just can't seem to get myself moving."

Therapist: "Fatigue makes it difficult to get motivated, which can help us to feel unproductive."

Client: "Exactly. Each day that I don't get anything accomplished, I start to feel worse about myself."

Therapist: "Knowing that you are going to feel discouraged seems like it's helping you want to give up . . . even before you get started."

Notice that the emphasis is staying on the client through their experience. There is no effort to advise, redirect, or interpret any feelings or behavior. Instead, the therapist believes their job is to stay with the client through their pain, helping them to feel less alone and more cared for. The idea is simple: give the client the emotional support they need without any type of judgment, and their own natural instincts will kick in to help them get on track.

OTHER ORIENTATIONS

Hundreds of other theoretic approaches are not mentioned; some are highly specific to certain populations, and others have broader application. Family therapy is an example of a broader classification of theoretic orientation, which emphasizes the system over the individual. Family systems theories, such as strategic and structural, emphasize the contextual elements and functional dynamics that impact individuals. In many cases the family is expected to be part of the therapy, while in other cases the individual comes alone but focuses on the various influencing systems in their life.

When considering which theory seems to fit with your own belief system, it may help to ask the therapist to explain how they see the theory working. Since most therapists are eclectic, their interpretations of the theories that inform their approach may differ from the conceptualization of the original theory. What's important is that if you want a more interpersonal therapy that emphasizes the relationship between client and therapy, you shouldn't select a strategic approach or one that focuses on the past. If you want a more existential approach that helps you look deeply into the meaning of life, don't seek a therapist who is more support oriented.

Ultimately every therapist will have some beliefs that are enlightening and others that don't seem to fit your own paradigm. What's most essential is to have a notion of the way in which people change and what the role of the intervener is. Therapists who don't have any allegiance to an orientation may be more susceptible to aimlessness or unclear direction. A therapist who holds a strong belief system in one theory may be inclined to fit you into that perspective, as opposed to seeing you clearly as a unique being.

FEAR FACTOR (BY DEB R)

I am afraid of everything, all the time. This is a new revelation for me. I knew I worried a lot and often felt anxious about things that were going on in my life. I now realize that what I have been feeling isn't anxiety but mind-numbing, paralyzing fear. This fear has been with me for a long, long time, so I had become somewhat accustomed to living with this emotion. I found ways to escape it, deny it, and bury it, but I have never found a way to get rid of it.

On the surface, this fear of all things seems pretty ridiculous. I was never in grave danger or felt I truly had to run for my life to escape injury. Taken on an individual basis, these fears can be dissected and maybe even "put to rest." Taken as a whole, this fear is overwhelming and often prevents me from action of any kind. I have come to realize that, although self-preservation is instinctual to all human beings, this type of fear is a learned response. I was not born being afraid but became so due to influences in my life that I am just beginning to understand. If a dog bites a child, then that child becomes afraid of dogs. Parents of this child can affirm this emotional response by becoming overtly fearful themselves. They tell the child to be afraid of all dogs no matter what happens. "Run, run," they say, "when you see a dog." So, the child learns to run from things that scare them. They can, however, teach the child to be cautious and smart around dogs without instilling a phobic fear.

With that being said, I would like to let everyone know how I came to realize this "ah-ha" moment. I did not explore my reaction at the time but chose instead to deflect away from her revelation. I deliberately chose not to connect with her. Why? Because I was afraid. My marriage is the one area of my life that still remains very closely guarded. I believe we have a good marriage but after thirty years have fallen into a complacency that has begun to define us as a couple. We figure that what is working should be left alone, so we don't explore this large aspect of our lives very often. I have learned the quickest way to divert attention away from a subject that makes me uncomfortable is to disconnect by expressing the total opposite of what is being discussed. Period, end of discussion, shut that door real fast. I hope this week I can be more open to and less afraid of discussing the "M" word (marriage).

III

Practical Considerations

6

UNDERSTANDING MANAGED CARE AND HEALTH INSURANCE

For many therapists, managed care is associated with the bastardization of therapy, justifying treatment requests, constant battling for reimbursement, and unfavorable limitations and restrictions placed on therapy. It is for this reason that a growing number of therapists decline to work with insurance companies or have dissolved their existing contracts, making it more difficult for clients to access qualified professionals in a timely manner while accessing their health benefits.

Clients seeking therapy should prepare for the exhausting and oftentimes frustrating process of finding a therapist through their insurance company, if this is the route you to need go. The initial call to one's insurance yields several names, sometimes five to ten providers in your geographic region. Factors including gender, specialty area, and license type can narrow the search results even further.

Once the initial calls are made, it's common to get voice mails instead of live people, requiring you to leave a message. Many therapists don't call back, an unfortunate side effect of having very full caseloads and a disregard for good "customer service." For those few who actually answer the phone, many have waiting lists and/or are not accepting new patients. It is common for those with HMO plans to be given less priority, although few professionals may admit to this. With more therapists moving toward private pay as their only option for services, the choices for selection may continue to decline.

The therapist names your insurance company provides may in fact have a high degree of expertise in the area you identify, but oftentimes the insurance lists just read from a database that has check marks next to issues treated. If a case manager is making calls for you (something you can request), they are primarily interested in finding therapists with openings and not likely looking for other factors outlined in this book.

Making your selection based on the list of available practitioners is a challenging experience, contingent upon the saturation or scarcity of available resources. Approaching your search with patience and persistence will help you to not get discouraged.

Through the first list of providers given to you, you are not likely to find a therapist who is warm, inviting, attentive, interested, knowledgeable, inspiring, encouraging of self-exploration, and capable of providing a safe space to work. If you call ten therapists from the list your insurance company gives you, you can expect to have maybe four return calls. Unfortunately, even a therapist trained in sensitivity to people's pain may not call back to make an appointment.

When you do get therapists on the phone, only two out of the four therapists you speak with may have an opening that fits with your schedule. So your choice is often influenced by attrition, such as who are the last few therapists left on your list after all these calls are made. Admittedly, this is not an ideal way to find a therapist who is going to help you with the most serious issues facing you in your life.

Private payment for therapy has advantages, including an increase in privacy and no limits on the number of sessions. The issue of privacy has become important with the advent of electronic billing and dissemination of information. Although there is no hard evidence that using your insurance will jeopardize your privacy, clients regularly voice concerns about how secure their information is and the potential consequences of being diagnosed (a prerequisite if you are using insurance). The introduction of preexisting conditions may have first led people to question whether they wanted a formal diagnosis in their permanent record, because they wondered if it would interfere with securing new insurance when changing jobs. More recent concerns have to do with employers and whether the use of insurance will affect jobs. While there may not be many known examples of confidentiality being jeopardized through insurance use, recent incidents of large-scale data theft have left people wary.

Most people aren't aware that insurance reimbursement, or third-party payment as it is sometimes referred to, is based on a model of medical necessity. Many insurance companies will not pay for mental health counseling unless a serious medical condition is indicated, such as major depression, schizophrenia, or bipolar disorder, to name a few. This means that those with adjustment problems, such as relationship strife, are not always considered eligible for reimbursement or have different co-pays/fewer sessions available to them.

Therapists have worked around this issue in the recent past, stretching diagnoses to help their clients use their coverage. The danger with this strategy is that insurance companies routinely audit cases, sending clients for independent medical evaluations (IMEs). If a diagnosis has been applied inaccurately, the insurance company has the right to terminate services or, in some cases, request its money back. If this happens, the therapist may then seek to recover the lost revenue from the client. Imagine this happening after being in therapy for an extended period of time.

It becomes even more confusing to clients who call their insurance companies and get a list of therapists in their network but are not told about these limitations. The insurance representative answering the phone is not the one who pays the bills, and in fact the offices may be in different states. So don't rely on the person assuring you that services are available because they aren't likely to be aware of the diagnosis limitation.

WHAT INFORMATION DOES MY INSURANCE COMPANY HAVE ABOUT ME?

This is a question with growing importance in this digital era. Our personal health information is extremely private, yet strangers have access to this information at the push of a button. Stored in databases are logistical data you provide to your insurance company when you sign up for health insurance, plus every doctor visit, lab result, and medication you take from that point forward. A therapist is required to provide your insurance with additional data about your treatment.

This information begins with a diagnosis. All mental health professionals use either the DSM (Diagnostic Statistical Manual) or the ICD (International Classification of Diseases) to utilize codes representing certain disorders. Each diagnosis has a three-digit number followed by a period and then a couple of other numbers (e.g., 296.21 is major depression, severe, single episode). This diagnosis will be permanently embedded in your record and cannot be removed. It's important to consider whether you are okay with this prior to starting therapy, because it can have unknown implications later in life, especially when considering sensitive employment matters.

Following the diagnosis, the insurance company requires TRFs or OTRs, which are ongoing treatment request forms. Since you are approved for only a certain number of sessions at the onset, the therapist must request more sessions as time goes on and justify the reasons why. Some insurance companies require minimal information, such as the number of sessions requested and the anticipated duration of therapy. Others ask for detailed goals, medications taken, and other data about daily functioning.

In addition to what the insurance company asks for on a routine basis, it has a right to review your **entire treatment record** at any time during or following the course of therapy. This includes all the private progress notes that a therapist writes following each session. While many therapists attempt to keep these notes somewhat vague, it is impossible to be nonspecific while meeting the general requirements of record keeping.

WHY DO INSURANCE COMPANIES CONTROL THE NUMBER OF SESSIONS?

Most insurance plans have a limit on either the number of sessions or the amount of money afforded to you in a year. The better the plan, the more sessions you typically get. For instance, many HMOs may give you twenty to thirty sessions, whereas some PPOs provide up to fifty sessions in a given year. If you remain in therapy for a year, then you would estimate needing at least fifty-two sessions, which is one per week. Sometimes session limits vary by diagnosis.

When you first get a letter from the insurance or managed care company, you may see only a handful of sessions authorized. This does not mean you are limited to this number; it means it's the amount given at this point in time. Prior to running out of sessions, your therapist will send in a request for more sessions, which is reviewed and generally accepted in the first round. Managed care policies seem cyclical, in that no authorizations may be needed for a period of time until the procedure changes yet again.

It is a good idea to keep track of how many sessions you have used and not just rely on the therapist to keep track. Most therapists monitor this for you as a courtesy, but it is ultimately your responsibility, as the insured, to keep good records. If you exceed the number of sessions authorized, you may be responsible for paying your therapist's fee. The statement of understanding form most therapists have you fill out at the start of therapy makes clear who is responsible for authorizations.

If you do have to pay for sessions beyond your annual or lifetime maximum, the therapist is only allowed to charge you your contracted rate. This means the co-pay plus whatever portion the insurance pays for, as opposed to the usual rate for your therapist, which is always much higher.

WHO IS RESPONSIBLE FOR GETTING ME AUTHORIZED OR REAUTHORIZED?

This is an important question to ask at the start of therapy. We may assume the professional is the one who will track our sessions and get us continued authorization, although this is not always the case, nor is it always done accurately or in a timely manner. For initial authorization, ask the therapist who will be responsible for gaining authorization. If the therapist would like you to do this, here is a list of questions you want to ask:

1. I am requesting authorization for outpatient mental health therapy for _____. Do I need an authorization and can you tell me what my benefits are?
2. What is the authorization number?
3. How many sessions do I have approved initially? How many are available to me over the year?
4. Do I have a deductible? What is my co-pay? (Almost every insurance plan requires you to pay for a portion of the therapy.)
5. Is the provider I wish to see in-network? (This means the clinician has a contract with the insurance company.) For those therapists

who are not in-network, do I have an out-of-network benefit? What is the deductible and co-pay?

6. Where does the therapist send TRFs or gain ongoing authorization?
7. Where do claims get sent? Whom do the checks get sent to?
8. Do you work on a calendar year for renewing my benefits?

Always get the name of the person you are speaking with, since you can speak with three different people and get three different answers to the same questions. Having a record of whom you spoke with and when can help when disagreements need to be addressed.

After the initial sessions are used, the therapist may submit a request for more, or the therapist may have you do this yourself. Even if your therapist assumes responsibility for this task, it is important to track the number of sessions you have used. While therapists consider it a courtesy to get you authorized, mistakes and miscalculations are made, and the therapist holds you responsible for a session that the insurance refuses to cover.

If you know when you are down to a few sessions left in your authorization, you can remind the therapist that he or she needs to submit the TRF. This raises the likelihood that the therapist will absorb mistakes, and they will not be your burden.

IS MY THERAPIST IN-NETWORK?

Insurance companies establish contracts with providers in different communities to offer psychotherapy services to their consumers. Insurance companies have many requirements for participating clinicians, such as education, licensure, malpractice coverage limitations, years of supervised experience, and expertise in certain areas. Insurance companies require certain record-keeping practices, particularly around privacy, to ensure protection for clients.

The benefits to a clinician for being in-network are steadier referral streams and an established rate of pay. To access a list of providers in your insurance company's network, you can call the member helpline on the back of your insurance card, usually a 1-800 number. You may have to call back several times to get more names and numbers if you don't have initial success. You can even ask your insurance company for help in finding you a therapist if you are unable to find one yourself, saving you valuable time.

In certain instances, you may find a therapist to work with before you contact your insurance company. There is a chance this therapist does not have a contract with your insurance company and is considered out-of-network. This may not be a dead end if your insurance company (or managed care) offers out-of-network benefits. The insurance company can easily tell you this over the phone if it is the case, although benefits are different, meaning higher co-pays or a deductible.

When seeing a therapist who is out-of-network, the clinician may ask you to pay his or her fee and wait to be reimbursed by the insurance company. Clinicians do this because many insurance companies pay the client directly and not the clinician. It can take several weeks (up to two months) for initial claims to be paid, so prepare for this financially from the start.

The therapist will be submitting HCVA (billing) forms to the insurance company, which indicate dates of service, type of service (individual, family, group), and the location of the service (office). If you would like, the therapist can provide you with a copy of these HCVAs so that you can track what your insurance company has received.

It isn't uncommon to have to stay on top of your insurance company with repeated phone calls to get reimbursed. The company may indicate that it hasn't received the claim or that it wasn't completed correctly. This is standard practice for insurance companies, and the persistent client will handle this in a patient but determined way. You can always call upon the therapist to assist with this process. Because the clinician is saved from having to do the billing, he or she may be more willing to keep you as a client and help navigate the difficulties with insurance billing.

In some cases, there is no out-of-network benefit, yet you are determined to work with a certain therapist. If this happens, contact the insurance company, tell the company you have exhausted the list of providers it has given you (several times), and have the name of a therapist you wish to see. The insurance company can develop an ad hoc contract for your particular case. This is an agreement between the insurance company and the therapist to see you for a certain period of time. Although the strategy can require a fair amount of arrangement time, it may be worthwhile.

CHECK YOUR EOBS

An EOB is an explanation of benefits. Each time your insurance company pays or does not pay for services (following the submission of an HCVA), the EOB is sent, with or without a check, to the provider (or the client if that is the arrangement). It is important to check your EOB for several reasons. You want to make sure the insurance company has an accurate reflection of the sessions you have used to help you compare with your authorization. It is also a way to ensure that your co-pay hasn't changed.

Quite frequently an insurance company will change the amount of money you are responsible for paying without letting you know, or they wrote about it in a form letter that you have discarded. It is also possible that the person on the phone who explained the benefits provided the wrong information.

WHAT IS AN EAP?

Many large companies have EAPs, or employee assistance plans. These are outside agencies hired by an organization to provide all types of assistance, such as legal, medical, financial, psychological, and so on. EAPs are generally short term, used for assessment and referral. Before considering therapy, it might be helpful to ask your company if it has an EAP, because EAPs are free and highly confidential. It can be a helpful way to determine whether therapy is indicated.

If you use a particular clinician with your EAP, make sure they are either in your managed care network or their rate is reasonable so you can continue therapy when your sessions have been exhausted. Some EAPs do not allow for self-referrals, meaning you can't see the same person after the EAP, which is also a detractor.

COMMON INSURANCE PROBLEMS THAT SABOTAGE THERAPY

Billable Diagnosis

Insurance companies tell their callers that they have mental health benefits, and if they call the list of providers offered to them, they are eligible for therapy. What they leave out of this conversation is the important element of diagnosing. Since the insurance company works from a medical model, only certain diagnoses will allow for third-party reimbursement; that is, your insurance company paying for services.

It is common for a first-time caller or even somebody who has had therapy before to insist that they will be covered, because that is what they have been told or they have found success with another provider. The sad reality is that if all therapists were to accurately diagnose, many people would not be eligible for their insurance to pay. Because of the ongoing struggle between clinicians and managed care, diagnoses are stretched or even falsified so that the client can use their insurance. While this may seem like a generous act by the therapist, it poses several problems.

Misdiagnosis or "stretching" the diagnosis can result in trouble for both clinician and client if the insurance company orders an IME (independent medical evaluation). These are done to ensure that clients are receiving appropriate care, but also because insurance companies can save money by deciding that therapy is no longer indicated. If it is determined via IME that the original diagnosis was inaccurate and the insurance rescinds coverage, the therapist may be asked to return payments, which in turn would lead to the therapist to ask the client for those payments, potentially devastating a client who is struggling financially.

Thus, if your therapist suggests that no diagnosis exists to warrant therapy, recognize they may be seeking a more ethical stance that protects both client and clinician. Stress, marital discord, problems with children, and many other stressful situations we deal with every day may not be deemed "medically necessary" by insurance companies for treatment. When you are new to therapy and hearing one thing from your insurance company and another from the therapist, it can cause stress that you just don't need. Clients may go straight to doubting the therapist, in part because they don't want to hear that somebody else will allow them to use insurance but this therapist won't.

Or in some situations a diagnosis may not be clear in the first session or two. If you bring a client into therapy and don't decide for two or three sessions, what happens if the decision is that nothing billable exists? The client now faces the dilemma of whether to pay for what they already had out-of-pocket, go on paying for future sessions privately, or start over with somebody new with the same potential problem still out there. This issue can easily lead to a failed therapy experience with some not wanting to try again.

You can remind the therapist, however, that even if he or she doesn't find a billable diagnosis, they are still obligated to charge you the rate contracted with the insurance company. So if your plan pays $74 for a session (remember that first sessions are often more), that is what the therapist should be charging you out-of-pocket. This also helps you to know that the therapist is not looking to make more money but they are interested in being ethical.

Putting the burden of money aside, ask yourself whether you would want to work with a therapist who broke the rules and behaved unethically just to save you money. While it may sound tempting in the short run, this is someone with whom you need to develop a deep level of trust, so any doubts that arise may whittle away this important quality.

Coverage Limits/Exclusions

Knowing your particular coverage, including limitations/exclusions, is very important. If you don't know your own policy and leave it up to the provider, mistakes may be made and not caught. Therapist and client must work together as a team to understand the complexities of your policy and keep up to date on the changes that nearly always seem surprising and random. You must scrutinize your own policy line by line, and if you don't understand something, have it explained to you by your employer's human resources department or the department who purchased the policy. There is generally an insurance/benefits administrator at the top of the heap of "insurance officials."

Deductibles and co-payments/coinsurance often cause problems with regard to coverage limits and exclusions, not including diagnosis. For some, a deductible starts on January 1 of each year, while for others it's the date of policy activation. A deductible may combine medical and mental health, or it may not. A co-payment may be different after a certain number of sessions have been used, especially if the insurance company uses a percentage system. All of this can lead to a host of misinformation that confuses the client and could lead them to lose confidence in the clinician who is continually readjusting the amount owed.

The best plan of action is to be in constant contact with the billing manager or person responsible for dealing with the insurance. Learning this information may be time consuming, tempting you to leave it in the practitioner's hands, but the problem can derail therapy. Imagine owing hundreds of dollars more than you thought because the co-payment amount originally acquired from the insurance company was inaccurate. Checking your explanation of benefits can help offset this problem.

Insurance Companies Are for Profit

Insurance companies' job is to make money, not spend money; as a result, they do what they can to save money. This can mean denying claims for various reasons, limiting the number of sessions you have or the frequency at which you can use them, or even providing wrong information.

Insurance companies make rules, change the rules, and then change them again with very little if any notification to the providers and patients. Claims can be submitted but not "acknowledged" by the insurance company for various reasons (many unknown to the office submitting the claims) and then be denied for untimely filing. They have the checkbook, so basically they are in charge of how much is paid, whom it's paid to, and when. This can be distressing for a clinician who works hard to provide services and then has to wait months or years to be reimbursed, spending countless hours and money fighting for compensation.

There is all kinds of speculation about how insurance companies work to save money. An agent from a major insurance carrier (who only wanted to self-pay because they were afraid of what having a diagnosis would mean in their record) disclosed some of the tactics used to save money: losing claims, sending claims back as unpaid with arbitrary errors, paying only partial claims, and even using algorithms to automatically reject a certain percentage of claims. Insurance companies are simply too large with too much bureaucracy for a small practice to fight against, so oftentimes these claims are left alone, reinforcing to the insurance companies that money can be saved through these practices.

Coverage Limitations and Benefit Information

Along these same lines of coverage limitations, be sure to inquire if the modality of service (individual, family, group, couples, etc.) is covered. Couples therapy is oftentimes the tricky one, because rarely is it covered under that name; it is under "family therapy." Not relying on the therapist or the office to assure coverage leaves less room for error. If you *always get the name of the person you are talking to* and the exact quote of what they are telling you, it will be easier to appeal the problem later on.

Getting inaccurate benefit information, particularly patient responsibility (co-pay/coinsurance), seems to be an ongoing issue. Many times the office is told one thing, but the claims are coming back with something completely different. It's not unheard of to be told something different by five different people at the insurance company, especially if the payor company is not the same as the authorization company (managed care system). Even something as simple as the provider being listed as in-network may be inaccurate, so be wary. Sometimes the provider is listed by the company name as opposed to their own, adding to the confusion. And never assume that if one provider in the practice is in-network, the others are as well.

The bottom line for reducing the potential for failed therapy based on pragmatic issues such as managed care is being an active participant in the process. Communicate constantly with whatever office is responsible for billing and assume that mistakes will be made. Mistakes are frequently made, many of which are due to the changing complexities of managed care, so it's important to catch them as early as possible.

Interesting Facts

- Mood disorders such as depression are the third most common cause of hospitalization in the United States for both youth and adults aged eighteen to forty-four. [1]
- Individuals living with serious mental illness face an increased risk of having chronic medical conditions. [2]

- Adults living with serious mental illness die on average twenty-five years earlier than other Americans, largely due to treatable medical conditions.[3]
- More than 90 percent of those who die by suicide had one or more mental disorders.[4]

7

PATIENT RIGHTS AND RESPONSIBILITIES

Even though therapy is about feeling better and growing personally, it is still a professional relationship often with a licensed professional, bound by rules and responsibilities. It's important to understand what to expect so that you can protect yourself, rather than trusting that a helping professional will always protect your best interest. This doesn't mean you ought not trust the person you are working with, but it does mean that an educated consumer is more likely to minimize exposure.

WHAT IS THE COST OF THERAPY?

This is an important question, especially if you plan on being in therapy for an extended period of time. Whether you are paying privately or using your insurance, the fees for therapy can be wide ranging.

For private pay, the cost of therapy is largely dependent on the part of the country you live in, the experience of the clinician, and the availability of resources. Psychotherapy can range in cost, depending upon your location (urban areas tend to be more costly), the experience and educational level of the therapist (Ph.D.s tend to be higher than master's-level therapists), and the nature of the therapy.

Family and couples therapy are sometimes more costly than individual and certainly group therapy. Private practices are generally more expensive than clinics because the professionals providing the service have greater overhead. Clinics and social service agencies tend to use students and less-experienced clinicians (although this is not always the case).

A doctoral-level therapist may charge a range between $85 and $250 per hour. The average tends to be around $150 per hour, increasing as you move outward toward the East and West Coasts. Many practices use sliding fee scales, making therapy more affordable. A sliding fee scale can be done in many ways but is most often based on income. Other practices have set fees ranging from $25 to $85, which include student therapists (interns), nonlicensed clinicians, and licensed therapists who opt not to be part of an insurance network or are not eligible to be in one.

DOES MORE EXPENSIVE MEAN BETTER?

More expensive does not necessarily mean better, and neither does less expensive mean worse. There are wonderful therapists who charge less money for many reasons, including the idea that they don't want to work with insurance companies and will reduce their fee to attract clientele who do not want a higher-priced clinician. It is likely that a therapist who charges a substantial amount of money has a good bit of experience and/ or has attained advanced training and/or accreditations.

There are institutes that offer specialized training to psychologists, including the Gestalt and Psychoanalytic Institutes around the country. These specialized clinicians may be worth a higher fee. The benefits to working with a therapist in training are numerous. They are often hardworking because they feel a need to prove their value, they are more accessible, and they have a more experienced supervisor in the background lending their expertise. For less complex issues, this can be a helpful savings.

WHAT IS A CO-PAYMENT? WHAT IS A DEDUCTIBLE?

If you are using your insurance to pay for therapy, you will likely be responsible for a percentage of the contracted rate, much the same as if you visit your physician or purchase medication. The amount of your co-pay is predetermined, although it can change during the term of the therapy, even if your insurance doesn't change. Some policies have graduating co-payments, such as $0 for the first two sessions, $10 for sessions three through ten, and $25 for sessions eleven through thirty.

You will be responsible for this payment at either the start or the conclusion of each session. You can usually pay with either cash or a check; however, more clinicians now accept credit cards. Having your check made out at the start of the session saves time and allows you and your therapist to work together for the entire time of your session. Being responsible with your co-pay is important because it lets the therapist know you value your time and are honoring your commitment to the therapeutic contract.

Some plans require you to pay a deductible before the insurance begins to reimburse for therapy. This is more common in the better PPO plans because they offer you more sessions and less hassle about authorization. If your deductible is $500, for instance, you will pay out-of-pocket until this amount is met, estimating at least three to four sessions. Remember that this deductible begins again every calendar year.

When checking to see if you have a deductible, you want to inquire whether the deductible covers both medical and mental health. If it does, you may have met the deductible sooner. Some plans have individual and family deductibles, which means that more money out-of-pocket is expected for multiple family members.

Knowing what the therapist's policy is about missed sessions, how much notice is needed to cancel, what happens if the insurance doesn't pay, and everything else financial is helpful for avoiding future problems. Some people may be surprised the therapist isn't more "flexible" or "accommodating" with regard to appointments, hoping that compassion would nullify late, canceled, or missed sessions. Keep in mind that a rigid policy on this matter is important, because you don't want a therapist resentful that they could have met with another client had they had notice of your absence. Even though therapists are largely drawn to this work because of their desire to help people, they also need to earn a living and take care of themselves in order to stay in business.

HOW OFTEN DO I SCHEDULE APPOINTMENTS?

Most therapists schedule appointments on a weekly basis. This seems to be an adequate amount of time to assimilate the work from the last session and prepare for the work of the next one. Anything less frequent interrupts the momentum of therapy, especially if you are early in your work. Later in therapy, or in particular when you are winding down, you may likely move to every other week or ultimately once a month. Most therapists will attempt to make themselves available at another time during the week if a second session is needed.

IS THERAPY CONFIDENTIAL? WHAT IS HIPAA?

Limits on confidentiality are determined in part by the method by which you are securing services. For instance, a mandatory referral from an employee assistance plan is going to have more limits to confidentiality than would a person paying privately, coming on their own volition.

Age is another factor that affects confidentiality and varies from state to state. Although children and adolescents need to feel a sense of safety and privacy with their therapist in order to open up about important issues, the law dictates the extent of this confidentiality. Understanding these parameters early in therapy can help avert conflicts with the therapist about what information about your child's therapy is available to you. For parents who are divorced, the importance of state and federal laws may be even more important, in particular if you are engaged in a custody dispute.

Another privacy issue to understand has to do with couples who seek therapy. While one person in that couple may be the "identified patient" with regard to insurance, meaning that only one person receives a diagnosis to submit to an insurance company (there are no diagnoses for couple's issues), both people have rights of privacy. If you are a couple and you eventually decide to divorce, both parties generally have equal rights to the information (sometimes dependent on who the identified patient is according to the insurance record).

The Health Insurance Portability and Accountability Act (HIPAA) is a federal law that provides new privacy protections and new patient rights with regard to the use and disclosure of your protected health information (PHI) for the purpose of treatment, payment, and health-care operations. The purpose of this law is to protect the privacy of patients with the advent of online billing and other information sharing through the Internet. HIPAA only applies to those patients who are using their health insurance to cover therapy. This doesn't mean, however, that patients who are paying for therapy privately aren't entitled to privacy; it simply means that confidentiality is inherently safer because no outside agencies have access to their records and nobody other than themselves is authorized to review their information.

Here are sample passages from a standard HIPPA form to give an idea of how confidentiality is treated:

Limits on Confidentiality

The law protects the privacy of all communications between a patient and a social worker/psychologist. In most situations, I can only release information about your treatment to others if you sign a written Authorization form that meets certain legal requirements imposed by HIPAA. There are other situations that require only that you provide written, advance consent. Your signature on this Agreement provides consent for those activities, as follows:

- I may occasionally find it helpful to consult other health and mental health professionals about a case. During a consultation, I make every effort to avoid revealing the identity of my patient. The other professionals are also legally bound to keep the information confidential. If you don't object, I will not tell you about these consultations unless I feel that it is important to our work together. I will note all consultations in your Clinical Record (which is called "PHI" in this agreement).
- You should be aware that I practice with other mental health professionals and that I employ administrative staff. In most cases, I need to share protected information with these individuals for both clinical and administrative purposes, such as scheduling, billing, and quality assurance. All of the mental health professionals are bound by the same rules of confidentiality. All staff members have been given training about protecting your privacy and have agreed not to release any information outside of the practice without the permission of a professional staff member.
- Disclosures required by health insurers or to collect overdue fees are discussed elsewhere in this Agreement.

- If a patient threatens to harm himself/herself, I may be obligated to seek hospitalization for him/her, or to contact family members or others who can help provide protection.

There are some situations where I am permitted or required to disclose information without either your consent or Authorization:

- If you are involved in a court proceeding and a request is made for information concerning the professional services that I provided you, such information is protected by the mental health practitioner privilege law. I cannot provide any information without your written authorization, or a court order. If you are involved in or contemplating litigation, you should consult with your attorney to determine whether a court would be likely to order me to disclose information.
- If a government agency is requesting the information for health oversight activities, I may be required to provide it for them.
- If a patient files a complaint or lawsuit against me, I may disclose relevant information regarding that patient in order to defend myself.
- If I am providing treatment for conditions directly related to a worker's compensation claim, I may have to submit such records, upon appropriate request, to the chairman of the Worker's Compensation Board on such forms and at such times as the chairman may require.

There are some situations in which I am legally obligated to take actions, which I believe are necessary to attempt to protect others from harm, and I may have to reveal some information about a patient's treatment. These situations are unusual in my practice.

- If I receive information in my professional capacity from a child or the parents or guardian or other custodian of a child that gives me reasonable cause to suspect that a child is an abused or neglected child, the law requires that I report to the appropriate governmental agency, usually the statewide central register of child abuse and maltreatment, or the local child protective services office. Once such a report is filed, I may be required to provide additional information.

- If a patient communicates an immediate threat of serious physical harm to an identifiable victim, I may be required to take protective actions. These actions may include notifying the potential victim, contacting the police, or seeking hospitalization for the patient.
- If such a situation arises, I will make every effort to fully discuss it with you before taking any action, and I will limit my disclosure to what is necessary.
- While this written summary of exceptions to confidentiality should prove helpful in informing you about potential problems, it is important that we discuss any questions or concerns that you may have now or in the future. The laws governing confidentiality can be quite complex and I am not an attorney. In situations where specific advice is required, formal legal advice may be needed.

Professional Records

The laws and standards of my profession require that I keep Protected Health Information (PHI) about you in your Clinical Record. Except in unusual circumstances that involve danger to yourself and/or others or where information has been supplied to me confidentially by others, you may examine and/or receive a copy of your Clinical Record, if you request it in writing. Because these are professional records, they can be misinterpreted and/or upsetting to untrained readers. For this reason, I recommend that you initially review them in my presence, or have them forwarded to another mental health professional so you can discuss the contents. In most circumstances, I am allowed to charge a copying fee of 75 cents per page (and for certain other expenses). If I refuse your request for access to your records, you have a right to review, which I will discuss with you upon request.

Patient Rights

HIPAA provides you with several new or expanded rights with regard to your Clinical Records and disclosures of protected health information. These rights include requesting that I amend your record; requesting restrictions on what information from your Clinical Records is disclosed to others; requesting an accounting of most disclosures of protected health information that you have neither consented to nor authorized; determining the location to which protected information disclosures are sent; having any complaints you make about my policies and procedures recorded in your records; and the right to a paper copy of this agreement, the attached Notice form, and my privacy policies and procedures. I am happy to discuss any of these rights with you.

Minors and Parents

New Jersey law gives children of any age the right to independently consent to and receive mental health treatment without parental consent if they request it, and if I determine that such services are necessary and requiring parental consent would have a detrimental effect on the course of the child's treatment. In that situation, information about that treatment cannot be disclosed to anyone without the child's agreement. Even where parental consent is given, children over age 14 have the right to control access to their treatment records. While privacy in psychotherapy is very important, particularly with teenagers, parental involvement is also essential to successful treatment. Therefore, it is my policy not to provide treatment to a child under age 14 unless he/she agrees that I can share whatever information I consider necessary with his/her parents. For children age 14 and over, I request an agreement between my patient and his/her parents allowing me to share general information about the progress of the child's treatment and his/her attendance at scheduled sessions. I will also provide parents with a summary of their child's treatment when it is complete, if you request it. Any other communication will require the child's Authorization, unless I feel that the child is in danger or is a danger to someone else, in which case, I will notify the parents of my concern. Before giving parents any information, I will discuss the matter with the child, if possible, and do my best to handle any objections he/she may have.

Breaking your confidentiality is one of the most serious ethical violations a therapist can make and can damage therapy beyond repair. There are some very blatant abuses of confidentiality, but more often, the violation is more subtle. Leaving records out for a secretary to read, leaving a message on your voice mail that isn't private, scheduling you at a time when somebody you know is coming or going from the office, are all examples of potential disruptions to your trust.

When these types of issues arise, try to be direct and swift about addressing it with the professional. You can often tell from the therapist's reception of your concerns whether the issue is repairable. Mistakes are made, so remember that everybody is human, but the hope is that your trust will be paramount to the professional and restoring it will be their top priority.

In some cases you may feel as though your rights have been violated to the point where there is no negotiation. In such instances you have the option of filing a formal complaint with the governing board that oversees the professional's license. This may be the Board of Psychological Examiners (psychologists), the Board of Social Workers, or the board that oversees the professional counselors in your state. All attempts should be made to deal directly with the professional so that you feel more peaceful, unless the infraction is grievous or you feel unsafe in doing so.

IS THERE A SPECIALIST FOR MY PROBLEM?

The general public uses the term *specialist* differently than the therapists who are part of professional organizations such as the APA (American Psychological Association) or the ACA (American Counseling Association). The generic meaning as we have come to know it is somebody who focuses primarily on a particular issue, has extensive experience treating this issue, or has gotten some type of advanced certification/training.

According to the governing bodies of the APA and the ACA, a therapist must meet certain requirements before calling himself or herself a specialist. This does not mean, however, that a clinician is not highly specialized in the area you are seeking help with. A better question to ask the therapist is, "What degree of confidence/experience do you have in working with my particular issue?"

People seeking specialists are often experiencing difficulties with addictions (sex, drugs/alcohol, gambling); eating disorders; or are children, couples, or the elderly. These issues and populations do require a certain level of sophistication because the issues can be complex. It is not advisable to work with a therapist in a more specialized area unless that therapist can convey to you a sincere interest and capability.

Issues such as depression and anxiety are not always considered specialty areas, but some therapists do spend more of their practice working with such patients. Inquiring as to the percentage of patients with such conditions that particular therapists treat may be helpful, but don't use this as the sole measure of aptitude. Instead, you might combine this with other questions suggested earlier, such as orientation and therapeutic approach. In the next section, we will discuss specialty areas in greater depth.

The safest way to proceed is to interview the therapist prior to making an appointment to determine their competency, familiarity, and comfort level with the issues you want to work on. Finding out these matters after therapy has already begun frequently causes people to become disenfranchised with therapy. Even if it's embarrassing to talk about, ask the therapist to discuss their experience and their approach with the type of work you are about to embark upon.

Inside Out

Well I wasn't dreaming
One foot in the quicksand
As I stepped into the camera view
Ready to tell it again
Well I'm not really sleeping
Lost soul in the quicksand
You know I'm at a precipice, with a twist
Rollin out on camera
With a goodbye kiss
(And now) I'm . . .
Turning all the inside out
Turning all the inside out
Burning out the inside
Now I have a secret army
That burns like a supernova
And they help me blow the secrecy sky high
Yeah, I can't sit still for too long
I'm losing all my patience
I never could imagine this, a catalyst
Monumental change
Or a goodbye kiss
(That's why) I'm . . .
Turning all the inside out

Turning all the inside out
Burning out the inside
Doubt kills
More dreams than failure will
You will see the light
And hear these words again, my friend
One day, I will heal *and* thrive
There isn't any pain
That isn't worth the gain
So lean into the rain
Here's my wish for you
Open up a window, let me walk on through
Here's my wish for you
Open up a window, let me walk on through
—Tim K

Interesting Facts

- According to a recent study, people with psychotic disorders, bipolar disorder, or major depressive disorder have greatly increased odds of reporting difficulties in accessing care.[1]
- Approximately 20 percent of state prisoners and 21 percent of local jail prisoners have "a recent history" of a mental health condition.[2]
- Seventy percent of youth in juvenile justice systems have at least one mental health condition and at least 20 percent live with a severe mental illness.[3]
- Approximately 26 percent of homeless adults staying in shelters live with serious mental illness and an estimated 46 percent live with severe mental illness and/or substance use disorders.[4]

IV

Preparing for Therapy

8

BEFORE I BEGIN

PREPARING A TIMELINE

Before the start of therapy, it can be helpful to prepare a timeline, either mentally or on paper, of important events that have taken place in your life. This timeline can include events and experiences as well as reactions to what has happened. It can be especially helpful to include any symptoms you can recall and their degree of intensity. For instance, if you have been feuding with your spouse with increasing intensity and as a result have been experiencing sleep problems, try to document it with as much specificity as possible. For instance, using a scale of intensity from 1 to 10 can measure things such as mood. A scale from 1 to 10 with the high number representing strong anxiety, for instance, can give you a way of assessing whether your worrying level is increasing or decreasing. The same holds true for other emotions such as sadness.

January 15	Arguing for over 2 weeks.	Trouble falling asleep.
January 25	Emotional distance from spouse.	Waking up twice a night. Mood decline: 2 points.

KEEPING A JOURNAL

A journal is different from a timeline because it's a more personal way of recording your thoughts, feelings, and behavior around important issues in your life. In addition to being a good outlet for distress, a journal helps you keep a record of your experiences. Once you enter therapy, it isn't easy to keep track of progress while you're in the midst of your turmoil. A journal can also be a real gift to yourself once therapy is complete because you can look back over your accomplishments to your starting point. Many who have gone through therapy have transformed themselves so thoroughly that they may not recognize who they were prior to the work.

Blogs and online journals have become more popular because they provide the opportunity to keep the journal more private, or in some cases, more public. Getting feedback on your entries can feel supportive, and it is entirely possible to maintain anonymity.

WHOM DO I TELL? CREATING A SUPPORT SYSTEM

For many, therapy is a very personal experience that took time to decide upon. For some, the resistance to initiating therapy has to do with shame or embarrassment about "needing help." For those who have great pride and believe they ought to be managing their problems on their own, therapy can present an initial challenge to self-worth.

Telling those who are close to you in your life that you are considering/starting therapy may be difficult. You may believe it's nobody business and keep it to yourself, or you may be proud of the idea that you are taking this step and share it with anybody you trust. Most people range somewhere in the middle, telling a select group who have their best interest at heart.

There is no clear right or wrong with whom you decide to tell. If you believe judgment and criticism are likely, it may be best to hold off and discuss the matter with your therapist. If you are unsure about the reaction you may receive, you can always test the waters by asking what others think about therapy to assess their level of receptivity. The stigma of therapy seems to have faded considerably over the years, although this is more the case with issues related to stress than to mental illness. There is also a disparity for affluent communities, who seem to take pride in the idea of therapies; however, this is a gross overgeneralization.

If there is a chance that friends and family will be open to your decision to start therapy, it's a good idea to let them know, because you are going to need a number of things from your "support system" while in therapy. The same may hold true for your job, if of course you believe there will be support through greater accommodation as opposed to a breach of privacy.

First, you will want support while you are expending large amounts of energy excavating hidden aspects of yourself and getting in touch with often painful experiences stored in the body. Therapy can be exhausting, and it's helpful to have caring others who can recognize this hard work and incentivize you during the tougher times.

Second, it can be useful if others provide you with honest feedback from which you can broaden your awareness. Observations and opinions from those who know you help to reduce your blind spots or the realm of unknown that each of us has about who we are. Soliciting this feedback can be more effective if others know why you are asking it of them.

Third, you may wish to experiment with new behaviors that have come about through experiments designed during your sessions. If you are working on being more assertive, for instance, this change in related-ness will be more readily accepted if the subject is aware of what you are doing.

If you don't have a solid support system, which is often a part of why people seek therapy, don't be dismayed. Your work in therapy will be building this network with whom you can do all of the above.

Those with whom you do decide to share don't require details about your sessions. What you opt to share with friends and family will be more a reflection of what you need them to know in order to gain feedback that raises your self-awareness as well as to offer support you need around experimentation. If you have very personal and private information you share in therapy, it may not necessarily be important to discuss it with others.

People who seek out therapy to deal with past abuse, for instance, may not be ready to share with others, especially during the early parts of therapy. Ultimately, however, if sharing painful memories or embarrass-ing information about yourself is part of what scares you, then it's likely there is value in building the courage to disclose to others.

REPLENISHING SPENT ENERGY

As mentioned in the previous description of a support system, therapy can be hard work, with many ups and downs. Sometimes energy is built with grand insights and successful experiments, and sometimes you feel completely drained, stuck, or seemingly taking steps backward. Even the most constructive and successful work can be exhausting, especially if self-care isn't optimal.

Consider someone who is going to the gym for the first time in a long while and maybe has decided to hire a personal trainer. This person is going to be tearing tissue to build stronger muscle, expending energy to build endurance, and feeling overall pain in the hope of gaining greater flexibility. To accomplish these feats more easily, this person will need to provide his or her body with better nutrients for fueling restoration.

The same holds true for therapy. You need emotional fuel to keep yourself hydrated, in particular when tackling the deeper issues. Who you are and how you get your needs met will determine what outlets you find valuable. If you are a homebody, then you might rent comedies, read humorous books, or schedule the occasional massage. If you are more outward, then going out with friends or taking an exercise class at the gym may be helpful.

21st Century Castle

This ain't no fairy tale
No knight in shining armor
White horses drive freeways
Impatiently seeking
Dragons to slay.
The princess knows
How to play dress-up
And fall in and out of love
But does she know
How to rescue herself?
—Jennifer S

9

THE FIRST FEW SESSIONS

WHERE DO I BEGIN?

Once you have decided on a therapist to work with, even if that decision is tentative because you haven't yet met the therapist or had the opportunity to see if your intuition matches your experience, there must be a place to make the plunge. After all, you can't fully decide if a therapist is right for you without giving him or her a full picture of what's going on in your life.

After the initial small talk or icebreaking, you may begin to wonder whose responsibility it is to get you started. Do you wait to be asked specific questions, or do you introduce something particular? Do you talk about your past, or do you give an update on your current dilemma? Some therapists may make it easier for you by giving you some lead, while others will allow you to sit with your discomfort so you can take charge. There is no right way to begin, but know that you can ask for help if needed.

Because you may have spent some time on the phone discussing why you are seeking therapy, this may be a natural point to begin. Providing some greater understanding of your current situation can help the therapist formulate a picture of what brings you in and what you might be expecting. If you didn't talk about your concerns by phone, you might ease into it by describing your symptomatology, much like you are visiting a physician.

Most therapists will help you ease into the session by sharing something about themselves, talking with you about being apprehensive to normalize your feelings, or offering you feedback on how you seem to them. Small talk, as with any other new relationship, is quite natural.

Once you have described your current circumstance, the therapist may ask some probing questions to get a sense of some important areas, such as what your support system is, how long you have been dealing with this particular issue (to assess severity of symptoms), how the stress impacts you, and what you have done to this point to improve your situation. All these questions and similar ones give the therapist an idea of what keeps you stuck and how much damage has occurred to this point.

Toward the latter part of the first session, or perhaps in the second or third, you will begin to discuss your ideas of what therapy is about and how it may be of help to you. Goal planning is like developing a road map with a starting point and an ending destination. Where would you like to see yourself when we say good-bye?

LEARNING HOW TO BE A CLIENT

The first part of your therapy, parallel to assessing the therapist and your working relationship, is learning how to be a client. The therapist sometimes assumes or overlooks that a client knows what they are looking for and how they may go about getting it. A client sometimes assumes that the therapist is going to "get it" right from the start or that it's possible to launch into exploration of an issue prior to establishing some realistic set of expectations.

It's difficult to be a client in therapy, because you have to attend to your own experience and assess the potential value of the therapist while simultaneously catching on to the style, method, and process this particular therapist uses. In fairness to you, the client, how can you possibly navigate all this while holding on to the distress that likely accompanies you to the session?

An experienced therapist is aware of this to varying degrees and so recognizes the learning process taking place. What is therapy about? What is the therapist's role in the relationship? How am I going to be an active participant in my own growth experience? What are the pitfalls we may experience, and what may we do about them? These are just some of the questions that this book attempts to cover but that need to be fully explored in the session itself.

GOALS: HOW DO I SET THEM?

Some of the most important work in the early stage of therapy is goal planning. This is how the therapist and client get on the same page with a shared picture of the issues and agenda for the solutions. The therapist learns what is important to their client, how the client has been struggling, and what their vision is about what they can or would like to achieve, while comparing their own experience of the client and what stands out.

Generally speaking, clients don't always have a clear picture of their goals, other than to feel better, relieve symptoms, or resolve a pressing matter. They may know they wish not to be depressed, or to resolve their marital turmoil, or to figure out what kind of career they want to change to, but these may be a starting point for more concrete and specific goals.

Let's use a more common presenting problem to demonstrate how goal planning is accomplished. A client, Mary, comes to therapy reporting a moderate level of depression. Upon investigation, it is found that Mary isn't sleeping well, she continues to gain weight, her marriage is stale, her career is not satisfying, and she is generally confused about her identity. So what might simply be diagnosed as depression has a mixture of ingredients, any one of which can be turned into a concrete goal.

Mary would like to improve her sleep, improve her self-image through better fitness, make some decisions about how to improve her relationships and her job, and so on. Goals such as these can be further broken down into measurable objectives. It's one thing for Mary to say she wants an improved body image but quite another to say that she will go to the gym three times a week, find a nutritionist, and discover the underlying reasons she has put the weight on in the first place. More behaviorally oriented clinicians will encourage specific and concrete objectives.

This last objective outlined for Mary, understanding the underlying reasons for her distress, is quite significant but more difficult to measure. Knowing *what is* helps us to appreciate the forces for sameness or the resistance we have to making a change. Mary may be keeping this added weight on for a variety of reasons, such as self-protection, avoiding the attention of males, or self-punishment for believing she isn't deserved of happiness. The key is learning the reasons for *what is* before attempting to make something different.

Any attempt at goal setting may begin with an appreciation for *what is* currently. You are having marital problems, so let's get a better appreciation for how these problems came to be. Did you start off attracted to your partner because he seemed strong and independent, but now you feel unnecessary? Solutions can be found in better understanding the problem, which means holding off on setting concrete goals too soon, or at least appreciating that they may change along the way.

Oftentimes the key to finding how to effectively get our needs met lies in knowing how we inhibit ourselves. This, too, comes under the heading of understanding what is. Once we gain this appreciation, we may sometimes decide we need to accept who we are and not try to make a change. If Mary can truly love herself for having a larger frame than her friends, maybe she can free up energy needed for other areas.

Sample Goals

A next step in therapy, after learning the basics of being a good client and deciding that the therapist and you are a good fit, is designing specific goals. Goals serve as a roadmap for therapy, helping you feel like you have a rough destination in mind. Some change processes focus more on how you are getting to where you are going than on a specific outcome, so don't get hung up on having a clear outcome if this isn't apparent.

Your wants, needs, and preferences will be used to develop your goals (broad, long-term) and objectives (specific, concrete, and measurable). Keep in mind that your goals are going to be expanding, sharpening, and even changing over time. The idea of goals is to help you envision the future rather than be prescriptive about what needs to be.

When creating this plan for action, remember you can and will make changes, so don't get caught up in making it perfect. Keep in mind that transformational change means that goals may be difficult to define, continuously evolving, and a negotiation between therapist and client. Some therapists aren't in favor of having a concretized set of goals, believing this is too narrowing and restrictive for what may be.

Oftentimes the process of deciding on goals is a negotiation with the therapist, who sees things that are in your blind spot. It's not for the therapist to tell you what is important, but it is helpful to expand your awareness when somebody points out things you may have missed.

What a therapist sees as figural (important) for their client comes from a mixture of places, including their theory or philosophy of life and change, their sense of what is hidden to you, their experiences with others who have had similar or related issues, and other intuitive factors. Therapists have mixed reactions to the idea that they hold an agenda for a client; some believe they attend only to what comes up at that moment in the here and now, while others work from a construct that guides them well in advance of each person they see.

The difference is that one therapist has the client inform the theory and the other has the theory inform the client. This means that some therapists will fit clients into their paradigm of what needs to happen in order to feel better. If you are anxious, then you need to do breathing exercises, guided imagery, and go to the gym three times a week, without looking at the underlying causes of the anxiety.

The plan developed below is an amalgamation of ideas used with clients seeking therapy for substance abuse. The key factors for each client to work on are stated at the top with a description of the work, followed by sample goals and objectives. These objectives may have relevancy even for those not dealing with substance abuse. The idea is to give you an idea of what a plan might look like, in this case for somebody with a substance abuse issue. Not every goal is used for the same client; it is a collection of common objectives based on many clients with the same issue.

Resiliency

An alternative but less-known philosophy of help for those struggling with substance abuse/dependency is most clearly articulated in a book called *Getting Beyond Sobriety*. Author Michael Clemmens describes an interruption to the cycle of experience in which people take actions not based on their needs but on their discomfort.[1]

If someone sitting on an airplane begins to perspire, tenses up their shoulders and neck, breathes more shallowly and quickly, all outside their awareness, they may instinctually ask the stewardess for an alcoholic beverage. This person is taking an action not based on their awareness of needs or the threat of unmet needs, but instead upon their difficulty sitting with their disease.

Sample Goals: Build a greater tolerance for distress.
1. Spend one meal a week attending to your sensory experience.
2. Learn a breathing technique which brings the body into greater contact with your other parts.
3. Delay gratification under duress for longer periods of time, such that the body learns that strain will not lead to decompensation.

Family Systems

Many people entering therapy have significant impairment in their relationships, family ones in particular. These ruptured relationships leave us feeling isolated and sometimes untrusting, which leads us to insulate ourselves even further. Exploring the dynamics of both past and present within these important family relationships can help illuminate unproductive patterns. Once we identify these patterns, we can work toward experimenting with more productive ones.

Some family dynamics include rigid or diffuse boundaries, another way of saying that we felt very distant or overly detached from our parents. We also learned how to express feelings, what behaviors were acceptable, and how to protect ourselves from real and perceived threats, all of which influence our current relationships.

Sample Goals: Learn how your family has impacted your addiction.
1. Have at least one family therapy session with your therapist.
2. Read an article or a book on relationships (e.g., *Codependent No More* by Melody Beattie or *Getting the Love You Want* by Harville Hendrix).
3. Write a letter to your family, taking responsibility for your addiction.

Relapse Prevention

From the moment you enter therapy, you are planning for your life without drugs, alcohol, sex, gambling, food, or other substance. Due to the ongoing risk of relapse or retreat into an early stage of coping, you may formulate a plan to reduce the likelihood of regression. Consider the tools you will need to develop and maintain a realistic plan for relapse prevention as you develop your plan.

Sample Goals: Develop a comprehensive relapse plan.
1. Learn to use retroflection, which is a skill for reducing impulsivity.
2. Develop aftercare support such as the continuing care group (once a week).
3. Establish a "home group."

Triggers

An important aspect of your relapse prevention plan will be identifying your triggers for relapse. A trigger can be a person, place, thing, or event that elicits certain thoughts and feelings leading to addictive behavior. Developing awareness of these "people, places, and things" will help you restructure your life in a way that minimizes your risk for relapse. You will also work to understand your internal and external triggers and, in time, develop strategies to provide you with strength for dealing with them.

Sample Goals: Increase awareness of triggers.
1. Make a list of people, places, and things in need of changing.
2. Keep a journal of thoughts, feelings, and behaviors influencing cravings.
3. Contact your therapist or group member at least once a day.

Self-Image

Most people who enter therapy have significant impairment with self-worth. Some may feel worthless, insignificant, and indifferent and experience self-loathing. Others may not yet have felt this pain and instead are holding on to a façade of themselves, which inhibits real honesty. In either of these scenarios, people will learn how to take a personal inventory, allowing themselves to genuinely assess who they are and who they would like to be.

Sample Goals: Improve happiness and self-worth.
1. Complete a personal inventory, which you may choose to share in group.
2. Read an article or a book on body image and self-esteem (e.g., *Like Mother Like Daughter* by Debra Waterhouse).
3. Complete a focus group on a topic such as assertiveness training.
4. Schedule an individual therapy session.

Thinking

Addiction is significantly impacted by our cognitions. The way people think about their use of alcohol or other drugs is a direct result of their thought process. It might be believed that if someone holds a job or has a family, they "couldn't possibly be an addict." This type of thinking is a way of protecting ourselves from the discomfort of dealing honestly with our problems.

During your goal-planning stage of therapy, consider what routine thoughts go through your mind and how "positive" and "negative" they are. Do you have negative thoughts that affect your self-worth? Do you have angry thoughts that affect your relationships? Is your rigid thinking preventing you from hearing feedback? The brain is like a tape recorder in that new messages can be taped onto our brain to play over the old ones. People can therefore learn to identify their cognitive distortions and restructure their thinking.

Sample Goals: Learn how your thinking affects your addiction.

1. Complete a worksheet on cognitive distortions (thinking errors).
2. Ask for feedback from three people regarding your thought process.
3. Keep a journal of thought replacement activities.

Relationships

If people can learn how to build satisfying and productive relationships, they will find greater happiness and reduce their isolation. Group therapy is a perfect opportunity to learn about oneself through feedback and to practice new behavior. One can practice effective ways of resolving conflicts, learn how to effectively share thoughts and feelings, understand how support is achieved through giving and receiving feedback, and ultimately learn how to ask for what he or she needs.

Sample Goals: Understand and/or improve quality of relationships.

1. Practice giving and asking for support/feedback in each group (required).
2. Engage at least one couples counseling session.
3. Read an article or a book about relationships.

Coping Skills

Oftentimes, people will turn to drugs and alcohol when their life stresses seem overwhelming. A primary goal for therapy will be developing tools for effectively dealing with internal and external stress. This may be stress management, relaxation training, anger management, or assertiveness training. It is in your interest to identify the tools you will need to effectively cope with life outside of treatment.

Sample Goals: Develop new coping skills.
1. Complete a focus group on anger management or relaxation training.
2. Learn a strategy for decision making and complete a practice exercise.
3. Complete a workbook assignment for anxiety or depression.

Improved Tolerance for Distress

There may be no more important or universal goal for people in therapy than to improve their capacity for distress. With a higher threshold for discomfort, we have greater room to make decisions, we will be less impulsive, we won't likely resort to less healthy outlets, and we will be more peaceful in our everyday lives.

We are motivated by both the avoidance of displeasure and the seeking of pleasure. When avoiding displeasure is our primary motivation, we give way to fear. We avoid risk taking that's necessary for making gains, we cut off contact vital to building energy and intimacy, and we live in a constant state of apprehension.

Sample Goals: Improve tolerance for distress.
1. Wait an extra five minutes beyond normal response time to stimuli.
2. Explore physical sensations associated with distress by writing them on paper.
3. One time during the day, replace smoking, drinking, and so on with meditation.

Resistance

Each person enters therapy with a certain level of discomfort, uncertainty, and reluctance, which can reduce the usefulness of therapy. Reluctance to accept the potential value of new ideas may be the single greatest obstacle to recovery. Those who enter therapy with higher internal motivation—

meaning they refer themselves or come willingly—are at a greater advantage than those who are doing so for somebody else (externally motivated). In either case, it is important to find ways of making therapy useful; otherwise, you will hurt others who are working hard to improve themselves. One of the first universal goals for therapy can be learning how to take in feedback to increase your self-awareness.

Sample Goals: Understand and decrease resistance to change.
1. Ask for feedback at least one time per group about your resistance/acceptance of treatment.
2. Identify which defense mechanism you employ through the use of a daily journal.
3. Establish a treatment plan you review each day.
4. Complete a resistance worksheet handout.

Support Systems

When people seek therapy, they are taking a risk in acknowledging that they don't have all the answers and don't want to continue trying to get well alone. It is instrumental to recovery to feel supported by others who understand and accept you without judgment or condition.

Sample Goals: Improve the scope of your support system.
1. Attend at least three AA/NA meetings per week (required).
2. Contact your sponsor at least one time per day.
3. Confide in a trusted friend or family member about your addiction.
4. Develop relationships with three new people with whom you can give and receive support.

Socialization

Enjoying oneself, whether alone or with friends, is vital to one's well-being, both during and after the conclusion of therapy. For many who suffer with addictions, there is an absence of "sober fun" activities to take part in. A useful goal for therapy is developing recreational interests that do not include drugs or alcohol. AA/NA meetings are a good place to meet others who have already done work in this area and may be a good resource for you.

Sample Goals: Develop sober social support and activities.
1. Develop a new hobby or interest to pursue daily, weekly.
2. Join the PTA at your child's school to make new friends.

3. Volunteer your time for an agency such as Big Brothers Big Sisters or a nursing home.

Health and Wellness

Caring for oneself is a task that many do not prioritize in their lives. In addition to the physical toll of drugs and alcohol on the body, balanced eating, regular exercise, and spiritual growth are often disruped. During your treatment goal planning, consider how you will reorganize your life to make this a priority.

Receiving a physical from your primary care physician inclusive of blood work is a good start. We may be lacking in essential nutrients and vitamins that can aid in our recovery. Improving our nutrition by removing GMOs (genetically modified organisms), eliminating processed foods, removing toxins in our environment, and increasing our intake of fresh fruits and vegetables can be a simple way to improve health.

Sample Goals: Attain a balance of physical wellness lifestyle habits.

1. Join a gym.
2. Exercise on a daily basis.
3. See a nutritionist/develop a diet of healthy foods.
4. Go visit a massage therapist.
5. Join a smoking cessation group.

Internal/External Conflicts

There is growing awareness through the early and middle stages of therapy that we are experiencing conflicts both within and between others that keeps us feeling tense. If we sacrifice internal peace by reducing external tension (giving in to others), we are likely going to feel restless, agitated, and even depleted.

Looking inward to find underlying unresolved issues affecting your recovery, either from the past or present, is helpful. Internal conflicts have likely led to confusion and ambiguity in your life, pushed away because closure didn't seem possible. You may not be aware of what these issues are, but with a willingness to explore, you may identify these areas that need closure.

Sample Goals: Identify personal areas of disharmony and gain closure/resolution.

1. Identify at least one unresolved issue and understand how it affects your addiction.
2. Find closure regarding a traumatic event from your past.
3. Learn how to balance personal wants/needs versus expectations from others (i.e., develop assertiveness).

Grief and Loss

Many are unaware of how loss affects them, even loss that is well buried in our past. Some are also unaware of what constitutes a loss and how normal it is to go through the stages of grieving. While in therapy, explore issues of loss, whether they relate to death, separation, identity, lifestyle, career, or something else.

When we do not effectively deal with issues of abandonment and loss, we often reinforce our unhealthy coping mechanisms such as alcohol or other drugs. Group therapy is a safe environment to examine these issues and find how to gain closure.

Sample Goals: Understand the losses in our life and find ways of feeling whole.

1. Learn the stages of grief and how you personally experience loss.
2. Read an article or a book on the process of grieving.
3. Gain support while working through losses in your life.

CAN I CONCEIVE OF TELLING A THERAPIST MY INNERMOST SECRETS?

We all have feelings, fantasies, experiences, drives, instincts, thoughts, traits, and so on that cause us shame and embarrassment. We keep them hidden so we don't risk ostracism that comes with feeling exposed. Keeping them hidden, however, can lead to fragmentation, as was discussed earlier. Even if we pay attention to these undesirables at times, we tend not to share them with others. Now, in therapy, we come to find out that in order to get unstuck, we must consider sharing these things out in the open.

To help ease your burden, consider that your therapist has likely heard many very similar or related admissions from other clients. After all, people have many commonalities, so it's likely that what you share will not shock a therapist. In fact, a therapist is likely to be impressed with the risk taking, revealing very intimate aspects of your personhood. Also consider that your relief from sharing such things out loud with another human being can be like lifting a huge weight off your back.

Remember that there is no need to disclose too much too soon. Instead, you might share with smaller risks and see how that works. If you share something slightly less personal and it seems to be okay, you may graduate to issues of greater substance. The only time restraints on therapy are the ones placed by you (and perhaps your insurance company). In other words, pace yourself with self-disclosure.

Also keep in mind that shame is a powerful barrier to healing, so if you are keeping hidden certain aspects of yourself, those are the limits to wellness.

IS MY THERAPIST SUPPOSED TO GIVE ADVICE?

This is a very difficult question to answer because there are no absolutes, and certainly there will be little agreement if you interview several hundred therapists. Different situations call for different approaches to working with a client, so how much you are talking is generally going to determine the balance of the conversation.

Therapists who are self-aware and put your agenda first are going to take their cues from you. If it seems you are having a difficult time knowing what to say, the therapist may talk more, or, conversely, if the therapist senses your need to vent, he or she may remain quieter. Remember that you can influence this by being direct with the therapist about what you need from him or her.

Regarding advice giving, this is slightly less ambiguous. Most therapists will tell you they are not the experts of your life, so how can they propose to tell you what is best for you? They may even tell you that giving you advice creates a dependency on the therapist that is the opposite of self-reliance, the ultimate goal of therapy.

Unfortunately, a large percentage of therapists will do just the opposite, offering their opinion often, believing their expertise gives them permission to influence your decisions through direct advice. Over time, therapists become lazy and look to rush solutions, leading to overdirection. While the occasional suggestion isn't harmful, a session full of "shoulds" and "ought-tos" defeats the purpose of therapy.

A therapist who is being genuine will have honest reactions to your situation and will sometimes decide to share them. Authentic therapists will offer you their immediate reaction to what you are sharing, which may be the closest many will come to offering advice. If you remain in a marriage where you are verbally abused, claiming that separation would be hard on the children, a therapist may point out that staying married may be even worse for the kids. So we can call this advice or just broadening one's perspective, although the difference can be murky.

Advice is a more superficial way of interacting. When we advise somebody, we are telling them what we think, what we believe, what we know to be right. This is limiting because it doesn't take into account our own biases, nor does it offer the other person your truest reaction. Here is an example from a group therapy session to illustrate this point.

One day a group member announces that he no longer wants to attend group and will be making this his final session. The group is initially stunned by this announcement and proceeds to ask questions about why he is choosing to leave. Initial responses include statements about a lack of time, difficulty getting out of work, the cost factor, and so on. Members begin to give suggestions about what this person might do to deal with some of the problems, such as making up work on different days and cutting back in other areas to afford the cost of therapy. All of these suggestions are waved off or dismissed with increasing ambivalence.

The therapist suggests that the member doesn't seem interested in a logistics discussion and encourages the group to share their feelings. One particular woman shares how sad she is that this person is leaving and how he has been instrumental in supporting her work. She believes she hasn't given enough back. From this the departing member explores how he has felt stuck and resentful that others hadn't noticed how much he was giving and not receiving. After a short while the member decided that staying in group was what he really wanted.

DOES MY THERAPIST JUDGE ME?

While we are told not to judge from an early age, most of us fail at this task. Realizing that judgment is a very natural and common way of relating can help us appreciate the starting point this gives us. Judging is believed to keep us safe because we are sizing up others to decide what threat they may pose. While we are not doing so intentionally, a portion of our mind functions as a self-defense mechanism. Who is a potential threat and who is an ally? Judgment is the mechanism by which we make these decisions.

The problem with judgment is that it's a fairly superficial means of self-protection because it shields people from better understanding themselves. Judgment is, in fact, as much about the person having the impression as it is the other. Here is an example: Pete judges Dawn to be rigid and controlling. If instead of judging her, Pete decides to explore what is being touched off for him, he may find that he himself is so flexible that he resents Dawn for the firmness of her beliefs.

So rather than viewing judgment as an evil we have to stay away from, we can view it as a way of learning more about ourselves. In this explanation, it may also be concluded that therapists judge because they are human. The difference is that therapists are trained to look beyond this superficial method of relating and into something deeper. They use the information about how they are reacting to their clients to better understand them. After this becomes more instinctive for experienced therapists, judgments are more seldom, replaced by a deeper appreciation for how they experience their client. The therapist's best tool is their sense of self.

HOW WILL I FEEL FOLLOWING THE INITIAL SESSIONS?

Forty-five minutes to provide a picture of your current circumstance and some background on who you are and where you have come from doesn't leave much time for deep work. For this reason your expectations of the first few sessions might be measured accordingly. You may leave the session feeling a sense of relief from having shared your story with another person, and you may even feel somewhat hopeful that you are taking action to improve yourself. Some people, however, may be so eager to feel better quickly that they leave the first couple of sessions discouraged because nothing is different. So, in short, how you feel following your initial sessions will likely be commensurate with your expectations going into therapy.

Some clients report feeling relieved that they were able to take this initial step. After the first session is over, they go home and assimilate all the information about the therapist, themselves, and the process of therapy itself. A simple yet complicated step of taking action to get help can be a powerful decision that alters one's sense of self. Try paying attention to what you experience following an initial visit and share it with the therapist in the next session. A therapist who is open to hearing your experience of him or her, yourself, and the process will help you to acclimate to therapy more quickly.

WHAT DOES IT MEAN TO CHANGE? WILL I BE A DIFFERENT PERSON?

The essence of who you are remains constant throughout your life—although experientially we grow as we learn more about life. Growing involves assessing our attributes and limitations to make decisions about where we want to build. Therapy does not change who you are or turn you into a different person. Instead, it assists you with the self-discovery process of finding lost or hidden aspects of yourself and then integrates them into your personhood. In essence, you become more of who you already are.

For example, a forty-six-year-old man, Joe, came into therapy because his wife and children had become so frustrated with his abrasiveness that they gave him an ultimatum of separation or counseling. Joe was baffled by their lack of appreciation for how hard he has worked in his life and the sacrifices he had made to provide for them, but he agreed to come to therapy.

Through the course of his work, he came to understand that he harbored resentment from giving up so much and not taking good enough care of himself, so he behaved grumpily around those people who didn't seem to acknowledge his effort. He began to create better balance in his life by reclaiming time for himself with hobbies and interests that were put on the back burner for many years. He took up woodworking and began to build items for his wife and daughters, which they truly valued. Ultimately, they built more intimacy into their relationships as Joe felt more whole as a person.

Joe didn't change who he was; he simply found a way to balance out the competing forces that left him feeling distraught.

WILL I HAVE HOMEWORK?

Because therapy occupies only a very small percentage of your week, the bulk of your work may take place in the days in between your scheduled sessions. When you are ready, you and your therapist may elect to design homework assignments. This may conjure images of high school and grades, but it is far from the case. For optimal homework assignments, you are both the designer and evaluator.

V

Multiple Paths to Change

10

THERAPY CONCENTRATION AREAS

CHILD THERAPY

When searching for a counselor for your child or grandchild, it is terribly important to find somebody whom both of you can trust. Finding that right person can be a challenge, so perseverance and patience are encouraged. It is particularly challenging to find a child or adolescent therapist who works with your insurance and doesn't have a long waiting list.

Working with very young children and adolescents can be viewed as two distinct competency areas, which may narrow the focus even further. Not all therapists are trained to work with very young children, who may require a particular modality called play therapy.

Play therapy is intended for young children who are not sufficiently verbal to benefit from traditional talk therapy. This approach has evolved since its creation by Virginia Axline many years ago. The most traditional version provides a safe and empowering environment that allows a child to feel in control (within reasonable limits). Through a technique called *reflection*, the therapist helps the child reconcile the conflicts, fears, fantasies, and potential traumas he or she may have experienced or is currently involved with. Some therapists will train the child's parents to do play therapy.

Other work with young children involves developing a language to express their feelings in a way that helps them get their needs met. Oftentimes peer conflicts result from low self-confidence, which affirmation and understanding can help. Involvement of the parents nearly always means greater success for a child in therapy.

Working with adolescents requires patience, persistence, and a willingness to meet them at their level. Adolescents often feel misunderstood and restricted in their lives. Some feel alienated, while others experience the pressure of their upcoming transition to adulthood. Common for this age group are eating disorders, cutting, and aggression. These behavioral anomalies typically involve a need for control, an escape from emotional distress, and a struggle for autonomy.

Interesting Facts

- Most cases of eating disorders can be treated successfully by appropriately trained health and mental health care professionals. But treatments do not work instantly. For many patients, treatment may need to be long term. [1]
- Eating disorders aren't just a problem for the teenage women so often depicted in the media. Men and boys can also be vulnerable. [2]
- Eat healthy foods. The frequent lack of adequate nutrients and presence of excessive fats, sugars, and sodium in fast foods can further sap the energy of depression sufferers. [3]
- Many may find that folate and vitamin D food supplements help improve their mood. [4]
- Some types of depression, especially bipolar depression, run in families. [5]

COUPLES THERAPY

Couples therapy involves three people—the therapist and the partners (a married couple, a couple who are dating but not married, or a couple who are divorced or in the process of divorce/separation). If it's a same-sex couple, it may be important to find a therapist in this case who is competent working with gay, lesbian, bisexual, and transgender clients.

Couples therapy differs significantly from individual therapy in that you are working with both intra- and interpersonal issues (within a person and between people) with an apparent focus on the latter. The client is the couple, though there may be one "identified patient" for purposes of insurance or record keeping. This is important to note in cases that may involve legal action. Generally speaking, release of records requires both partners' signatures, but this may vary by state.

Couples therapists work with their clients in two distinct ways. The first is to have the couple face the therapist, dialogue flowing through the professional. In this setup the therapist is viewed as the relationship expert who assesses and directs the clients more similarly to an individual session. This approach tends to be less threatening at first because the therapist serves as a buffer between the partners. In addition, this approach is designed to provide more interpretation and feedback about why the couple is having trouble and what they might do about it.

Many clinicians fall into a pitfall in this approach, which is becoming something of a judge to the couple. When two people are sitting across from the therapist, they may be tempted to plead their case, prove their rightness, or even wait for expert advice to solve their problem. If these things happen, the couple isn't learning how their situation developed and may be at risk of repeating the pattern down the road, even if their immediate issue is resolved.

The other approach is to have the couple face each other, and the therapist acts as a facilitator of contact. While this may seem more challenging to first-time clients, it offers the opportunity to better assess how a couple navigates intimacy. Having a couple speak with each other directly also approximates therapy more to real life. Instead of a contrived setting where clients look toward the therapist as a mediator, talking directly with each other better simulates what takes place at home. Additionally, this approach allows couples to experiment with new ways of relating to each other as opposed to going home and trying something new for the first time.

Couples therapy has two significant dimensions; the first involves mechanics. How effectively do the partners express themselves, and how well do they receive and convey understanding? How does the couple negotiate conflict and problem solve? Does the couple argue in a way that preserves respect/dignity, or is ongoing damage occurring? How does decision making occur, and how might the couple learn to compromise and negotiate more effectively? These and other, more functional aspects of the relationship are worked on through skill building and the development of awareness. The couple is taught to attend to the methods they use to get their needs met and how they might become more effective through improved communication.

The other dimension of couples therapy is identifying those issues that have likely created or at least reinforced the communication problems within the dyad. Although many couples cite "communication" as *the* problem within their partnership, oftentimes it is unmet needs which break down communication. For instance, if you believe your spouse has been insensitive to your need for reinforcement regarding your parenting, in particular because you are often saying how much you doubt yourself, then you may become resentful they haven't picked up on your clues. Instead of telling your partner what you need, you become quiet and withdrawn. Ineffective communication is the result of an unmet need in this circumstance and not the cause of your discord.

One of the first tasks in couples therapy is to help people balance looking inward and looking outward. The majority of participants are focused on what their partner has or hasn't done rather than their own impact on their partner. When both people are looking outward, they generate dynamics such as power struggles that prevent contact. We have limited power to influence another to do something differently, so we learn to appreciate our own potency, appreciating what may be impacting the way we relate. Improving our own awareness of the less-productive ways we try to get our needs met is a foundation to exploring more complex issues in the couplehood.

Many couples arrive at therapy with an identified problem, such as finances, sex, or communication, but they are unaware of the dynamics that led to this presenting issue. Differences in how finances are reconciled often involve power and control. Communication problems inevitably lead back to how needs are being met. Remember that what we identify as the "issue" is often part of the iceberg we see sticking out of the water.

Sex therapy is often a component of couples work, although sometimes it is addressed individually. If your therapist doesn't consider herself a "sex therapist," she may still have training and/or expertise in this area. The name can be misleading because it implies that this is a problem unto itself as opposed to an issue resulting from our intrapersonal and interpersonal baggage.

Strong neuropsychological interaction may be going on for those who suffer from premature ejaculation, erectile dysfunction, and difficulties with orgasm. The two components of the autonomic nervous system, the sympathetic and parasympathetic systems, are largely responsible for arousal and orgasm, working differently for males and females. This biological complexity makes it helpful to have a therapist who appreciates the mind-body connection and can be asked about it prior to or during a session. Many therapists will make referrals to a specialist if they don't feel comfortable doing this work, while others will engage with you freely.

Much of the work of sexual dysfunction comes down to what was described earlier, which is disconnection from our bodies. People who are highly stressed during the day, those who have had trauma, and highly intellectualized persons tend to suffer the most frequently. Very simply put, those who are in their heads make worse lovers because thinking has no place in enjoying sexuality. A therapist who is going to help you learn how to breathe and be more sensory focused will be most helpful.

Who brings it up? Somebody who is uncomfortable or doesn't see sexuality as the primary reason for seeking out therapy may be avoiding a potentially important issue. Similar to eating, sleeping, working, and playing, sexuality represents an important aspect of our personhood and an integral piece of our intimate relationships. While the therapist may inquire and hopefully does so to ease your anxiety about how this will get into the room, take it upon yourself to volunteer this information in spite of your worry. You will learn very quickly from doing so the comfort level of the therapist and the likelihood that this is a safe and meaningful topic for your work with them.

A particular way in which couples fail at therapy is when the therapist sees the couple after working with one person individually for a period of time. It may be tempting to bring in your partner to work with a therapist you have gotten to know, but the danger is twofold. Firstly, you may feel like you have lost your support system or confidant, because the focus is no longer on you but on the couplehood. More likely, however, is that your partner may feel ganged up on, or at least uncomfortable about the private matters that have already been discussed. Imagine walking into a room with someone you believe has already formulated an impression of you, and how tempting it would be to prove yourself or protect your perspective.

Another frequent occurrence when doing couples therapy is to work with each person individually while seeing the couple together. Sex therapists in particular use this approach to help each person get ready to address issues in the conjoint sessions. The risk here is learning information that one partner doesn't know and having to hold this information in confidence, without letting it influence your work. There was one occasion where a therapist learned of infidelity through this approach and then urged one partner to "come clean" before they were ready. This bred resentment in the therapy, which quickly became its demise.

Having clear expectations about what gets shared and what the restrictions are on privacy is important to prevent such occurrences. Even discussing who the "identified patient" is in the eyes of the insurance company, as managed care does not include any diagnosis for couples, will help prevent future problems.

FAMILY THERAPY

Family therapy generally involves at least one parent and another relative other than the spouse (both parents in therapy is generally called couples or marital therapy, unless the couple is divorced). For instance, it could be a parent and a child, a parent and a relative such as a grandparent, or even siblings who are working on their relationship. (Insurance companies do, however, refer to couples therapy as family therapy, because most don't reimburse for couples work.)

Therapists who utilize a "systems approach" believe that most, if not all, "problems" are the result of dynamics within the family. This is particularly important when considering therapy for a child. The temptation is to want the therapist to help the child without the involvement of the family, because it may mean dealing with very personal and complicated issues that can be uncomfortable to address.

The goals of family therapy vary, depending on the particular approach of the clinician and needs of the family unit. Typical overarching goals may include helping members identify roles, boundaries, subsystems, and communication styles within the family. In practical terms, this could mean helping children be more respectful to their parents, reducing arguments, and improving cooperation.

Roles are the positions we take up within the family that create our identity. These roles oftentimes satisfy a need in the family and help to create homeostasis (balance); for instance, an older child may become super responsible to help his or her parents, or a child may become the rebellious troublemaker to take the focus off something else in the family. What is your role in your family of origin, and how do you see this role with your current family and friends?

Boundaries, according to family therapists, are the invisible lines drawn around dyads that create subsystems. For instance, the parental boundary is the dotted line that separates the parents' relationship from the children. This boundary can be diffuse or rigid, meaning the children might be very able to involve themselves in their parents' relationship, such as the "parentified" child. A mother, for example, may talk with one of her children about her unhappiness with her husband (the child's father), bringing him or her into that subsystem. Boundaries can also be very rigid, meaning the children feel very isolated and cut off from the parents' relationship. "We never argue in front of the children" can be indicative of a belief that children must never know what's going on with their parents. Both of these extremes can lead to problems in the family.

Communication styles are the overt and covert ways in which messages about feelings, wants, needs, limits, and conflicts are expressed. Communication can be verbal or nonverbal, direct or indirect, clear or unclear, unidirectional or bidirectional, and so on. Learning effective communication patterns helps with resolving conflicts and negotiating differences more easily. Understanding communication styles can also help members build trust and intimacy within their relationships.

The therapist's role in family therapy is bringing all these concepts into focus so that members can better understand why problems exist. One of the first tasks of the therapist is typically to broaden the scope of why families come to therapy. For instance, there is typically an "identified patient," or a family member who is elected to have problems that make therapy necessary. A therapist may say to a family during an initial session that the difficulties described are the responsibility of the entire family, created by all the members and therefore needing to be resolved by all the members. This idea may meet with resistance from the one who doesn't see his or her role or want to acknowledge their part in the issue.

Once each of the family members considers this idea, the therapist will attempt to make contact with each, helping him or her feel understood and supported. The therapist will show they are objective without taking sides, even though somebody may come into focus first. This is important because many people who enter family therapy are fearful that they will become the focus or be blamed for the family's struggles. An ongoing process for the therapist will be to support the risks taken by each person and help the family while they become more balanced.

Throughout the course of family therapy, the clinician may call upon various members, including the youngest of the children, to share their perspectives about why problems exist in order to help each person have a voice. As fighting becomes more productive, defenses fade and greater closeness results. Children may feel less need to explode or implode, while parents learn to feel more potent. Oftentimes the parents will turn their energy toward the marriage, with the children becoming more peripheral.

Sometimes family therapy work involves adults and their parents, siblings, or extended family who may or may not be present for the session. The wounds inflicted during childhood may still be impacting us as an adult, in spite of the lengthy time which has passed since the trauma. In many instances our entire childhoods are marred by very painful experiences, such as being scapegoated continuously during our upbringing, blamed and ridiculed for events outside our awareness, or even injured through words and actions. While we may or may not call our experiences abuse, it is clear that we are suffering from overt messages that we were somehow not enough or not wanted by our caregivers.

In family therapy we spend time working through the pain of feeling inadequate and unwanted. We may work to address family members directly, or understand the way we have been shaped to relate in our own families. The way we parent our own children or select life partners is nearly always brought into the foreground to explore, so that we can both heal from old wounds and make sure that long-standing patterns are changed. In all family therapy work we require a therapist who can appreciate that our life involves systems, both small and large, which often get re-created in the image of what we have known.

A common threat to family therapy is confidentiality. If the family isn't seen each week at the same time, then questions will arise about what gets shared and what doesn't, especially depending upon the age of the child. Parents believe they have a right to know what is going on with their child and have a responsibility to raise that child in the six days, twenty-three hours, and fifteen minutes that they aren't with the therapist. Conversely, if a therapist loses the trust of the child, then no gains can be expected in therapy.

Addressing these parameters early and often in therapy can help avoid serious complications which can undermine therapy. Parents want to be informed and teens want their privacy, so this is not a new issue to the family; in fact, it may have been part of what brought them to get professional help. A therapist is responsible for laying the groundwork and helping to brainstorm these issues so everybody can be prepared. If the child is using drugs or having sex, what can they expect from the therapist?

Another issue to consider is what happens when the child doesn't want their parents involved with the therapy or isn't willing to have sessions together just to check in. If a therapist isn't following a belief that different professionals will be responsible for these different constellations (meaning one therapist for the child and another for the family), then negotiation is needed to prevent this from becoming a liability.

Along similar lines, what happens when family members decide not to show up for therapy? If a parent on one day decides they aren't interested or they "aren't able" to get their child to attend a session, what happens? This may be the case more often with divorced families where the parents aren't on the best terms. Depending upon the age of the child and the issue at hand, judgment calls need to be made to balance the best interests of the child and family, which can lead to resentment from any part of that system. For some clinicians who are more focused on the system, this may be seen as an important part of the family's work, and they may suggest postponing the session until everybody can be present. While this may seem harsh or punitive, it takes a very confident therapist to recognize resistance and value the importance of everybody being invested.

GROUP THERAPY

Group therapy can be one of the most exciting and rewarding experiences a person can have in his or her lifetime. If done well, it's a transformative experience that helps people to grow well beyond even what they themselves believed was possible.

Group therapy is a safe but challenging place that helps improve self-awareness. With increased awareness, we understand what helps and hinders us from getting what we want out of life while moving us closer toward fulfillment. Awareness includes appreciating your role, your interaction style, how you get your needs met, how you create intimacy/ distance with others, how you resist change, and many other insights about yourself in relation to the world. Group therapy is an exciting and supportive environment to experiment with new ways of being, getting/ providing support, discovering hidden aspects of yourself, and finding greater fulfillment in life.

There are two general types of group therapy—process oriented and content focused. Content-focused groups are more educational, and while they can be therapeutic, they are less likely to involve in-depth exploration of underlying issues. Process-oriented groups can involve most themes or topics, attracting people who are dealing with depression, anxiety, relationship issues, and almost every other theme imaginable. A specific kind of process group that we will explore more in this book is called experiential group therapy.

Experiential group therapy is vastly different from the types of groups you may have heard of, or even been part of. Instead of being content focused, as are most groups such as AA, grief support, and so on, these groups are process focused, an examination of the "how" as well as the "what." How do we get our needs met? How can I express anger without worrying I will hurt or offend? Experiential group therapy is a self-designed laboratory where you create experiments for improved relatedness.

In order for groups to be most effective, conditions such as honesty, consistency, receptivity to giving/receiving feedback, and a willingness to explore who we are in relation to others are all vital. Early in group it's difficult to make a full commitment, because we're not nearly versed enough to appreciate the full potential of this unique experience. Over time, however, as members work through their resistance, we come to appreciate the incredible gifts that group has to offer.

The Johari Window is a helpful way to conceptualize the value of group, as members become more aware of who they are through a balance of self-disclosure and feedback. Members move from safer, content-driven topics, building trust and cohesion, to more intimate dialogue around needs, using an appreciation of the group process as a catalyst. Nowhere else in our life can we so freely discuss how we manipulate one another or practice intense conflict, which takes personal growth to another level.

Issues of sexuality, fantasy, and identity are common themes explored in the later phases of group therapy. Members attune to how well we make contact with others, allowing us to feel more alive, more impactful, and even peaceful. Rather than getting lots of advice or suggestions on how to fix problems, people learn how others experience them through the issue. "I hear you talking about how your husband seems to take you for granted, but as you are talking I can feel myself doing the same thing."

We come to realize through group therapy that becoming somebody different is unrealistic and ultimately undesirable. Instead, we learn to come to terms with who we are while developing those aspects of ourselves that are dormant. People are often surprised that therapy is as much about self-acceptance as it is making changes to who we would like to be.

A significant distinction of a process group involves working in the "here and now"; in other words, it is of utmost value to attend to the dynamics of your exchanges, the experiences of yourself and each other in the room, and the role you are playing within the group. Through working in the here and now we will learn how to be more immediate, spontaneous, and authentic. The greatest opportunities for growth and the most rewarding experiences will happen when we are "in the moment."

To assist in determining whether group therapy may be right for you, consider the common goals suggested below. While this is not an exhaustive list, it will give you some appreciation of what members can expect to gain from the group therapy experience. Use these suggestions to generate your own curiosity and perhaps spark an interest in similar or related objectives of your own.

Sample Goals

Learn how to ask for support	Learn how to provide support
Experiment with new ways of relating	Increase self-awareness
Increase comfort with self-expression	Set healthy limits and boundaries
Explore similarities and differences	Improve decision making
Improve assertiveness	Resolve hurt and other painful emotions

Gain closure on unfinished business	Increase your overall sense of well-being
Understand your defensive structures	Improve intimacy within your relationships
Understand how others influence you	
Gain support and provide support to others	

Group therapy is a transformational experience! Members utilize their group experience to better understand who they are, gain greater self-acceptance, and create opportunities to experiment with change.

Your first few sessions may be filled with apprehension—wondering how others view you and how you will fit in, and trying to understand how the group works and how it might work for you. While there is no pressure to share when you are not comfortable, group is about learning to take risks. Coming prepared to share something about why you chose group therapy and what you hope to gain may ease in your transition.

In order for the group to become a safe environment to engage in important therapeutic work, a number of commitments are often asked of you: (1) arrive on time and consistently to each session, (2) be open and honest to the best of your readiness, (3) take risks when you feel safe and look for ways to create safety, (4) honor the work being done by others in the group, (5) keep all information confidential (including names and distinguishing information), and (6) extend the same respect to others as you would expect for yourself. If and when you decide to discontinue group therapy, coming to a final session to discuss your decision provides an opportunity for closure, both for yourself and others. Healthy good-byes are very important for closure and continued growth.

The therapist also makes commitments to the group: (1) begin and end each group at the scheduled time, (2) support group members in their efforts to grow, (3) encourage members to extend themselves as fully as possible, (4) challenge members to embrace new experiences, (5) support the generation of data, valid information concerning problems, (6) further the development of member skills in seeing new ways to work through problems, (7) help provide an atmosphere of safety, (8) enhance contact between members of the group and within each person, (9) be available to group members outside of the group should the need arise, and (10) become as marginal as possible.

Clients prematurely drop out of group therapy for many reasons. They may have hit a wall that they can't seem to get past; they weren't fully prepared for the challenges faced with real-life encounters; they may feel like they aren't able to make space for themselves, feeling more comfortable working one-on-one; or they were facing an issue with another group member that they didn't know how to work through.

When somebody is considering dropping out of group therapy, it's often indicative that important work is ready to be done. For those who stick it out and push through their ambivalence, certain growth nearly always seems to follow. If the group is safe from threat of harm, if the therapist isn't overly directive, and if the group members feel comfortable exploring their experiences of each other in the room, then it can be highly worthwhile to endure the discomfort that most certainly will arise many times throughout the course of your group work.

Client Experiences of Group Therapy

> I have been thinking about how much my perception of the "group experience" has changed since I first started. I realized this as I was thinking over the notes sent by Jared and how everyone responded on Thursday night. My first reaction was that of admiration and gratefulness for the honest feelings and emotions displayed by all of the members at one time or another. There was a time when I would have been very, very uncomfortable by this. Not only would I have been unable to conceive of the idea of doing this myself, but having others be so open and vulnerable would have made me shut down. (Even now I have a physical reaction when I say the word *vulnerable*.) I have really come to look forward to such honesty, especially from the newer members who are really taking big risks considering they have only known me for a short time. They have helped me by example and by allowing me to do my own work, sometimes using them as a springboard. My desire for this ability to connect becomes stronger and stronger every week. I am hopeful there will come a time when the desire for such emotional freedom will outweigh my desire for emotional safety and this will become my way of life. . . . I love you all so much.

Group is a sacred place. We have a circle of nine when we are all in attendance. We have grown, together, to trust each other. We nine know that we can bring in anything we need help with. And that if we aren't able to get what we need, we learn to ask for it. Jared sometimes has to do some leading, prompting, when needed. We have become powerful together in the hope that we can become powerfully authentic alone.

Group therapy is the place where it is safe for your walls to come down—walls you are not even aware that you alone put up. Other members have tools that they can lend you because they have used them. Some need them right back 'cause they are in the process of still bringing their own walls down. In many cases, it is a community project. Nevertheless, it is a "work-at-your-own-pace" place! I wish it were longer than 75 minutes.

Group has been a very useful tool for me. Like anyone else, I have had issues to deal with in my life. Group therapy has allowed me to recognize what they are and how to deal with them. Through group, I have come to the realization of other facets of my life having a negative impact on me and why I have not dealt with them, instead pushing them and hiding them away. Group has been a huge learning tool for me and has allowed me to grow and heal in a good way. Jared's guidance and knowledge has been valuable in allowing me to accept what I have to deal with and move forward in healing.

Group therapy is the safe and trusting place that I allow myself to deal with the issues I know I have, and the place that I discovered issues I didn't know I had. It has given me a place to experiment with relationships and real-life situations that I encounter. Group therapy has helped me grow into and to like the person I am today. It is the one thing that I truly do for me and no one else.

For the past two years my teenage son and I have been in therapy. His behavioral problems have been overwhelming at times and have put a cloud of doubt over my belief that my parenting skills are what they should be. I am a single parent and have no support from the other custodial parent.

When group therapy was mentioned to me I was excited to have a chance to listen and talk with others about "life events, feelings, and experiences." At first the adjustment was new and a bit different from one-on-one therapy, but understanding what you can get out of it is "real." The best part of group was not feeling alone. Even though some of the issues were different for each one of us, the sense of honesty, openness, and trust is what we all came to share. And the best part is also using these new skills outside the group with family, friends, and at work. It has given me a greater sense of trust in myself and a greater sense of self-esteem. I look forward to group each week because it is something that I do special for myself. One thing that I have realized is that I need to do for me so I can do for others.

Almost every week at group I learn I am not alone in my loneliness and that others struggle to find a peaceful place to be in their lives. When I hear others share their pain, the overwhelming sense of being by myself is lifted.

For me, this is about taking risks lately. It's not easy to let down the guard, to reach out to take those feelings buried deep and expose them. To search deep, to sort through the mess, and to see that I do have needs, and that I have not allowed myself to acknowledge them, let alone allow others to contribute to me. There is no great miracle in the moment, just a long series of small miracles there to be had if only one lets them come their way.

I have benefited from group therapy. Group helped me to focus on how I experience what I see, hear, feel, smell, and think—in short, how I experience what I sense. Group has helped me understand more about how I react, and what I do in reaction to experiences. Group has helped me focus on how my reactions are satisfying for me and limiting for me. How I experience group is more like how I experience daily life in comparison to individual therapy, and so I can pull from group experiences and relate them to everyday contact with others easier than applying what I learn from individual therapy. Group has helped me practice how I relate to others' points of view, especially my spouse's. My relationship with my wife has improved in every way since I've participated in group.

11

A WHOLISTIC APPROACH TO WELLNESS

The greatest mistake in the treatment of disease is that there are physicians for the body and physicians for the soul, although the two cannot be separated. —Plato

UNDERSTANDING WELLNESS

When was the last time you felt well? Not "well enough," or even "pretty good," but completely and optimally well? Sadly, we tend to measure health in terms of disease and/or discomfort. We base how well we feel on whether or not our allergies are acting up, how bad our arthritis is, or how intense our stress headache might be. In other words, we consider wellness the absence of symptoms as opposed to the presence of health and vitality.

We've come to accept minor, recurrent symptoms such as allergies and digestive trouble as part of the human condition instead of indicators warning us of compromised health. This chapter is designed to help you understand integrated approaches to wellness and prevention. It will help you become an involved, educated health-care consumer, ultimately raising the bar for your own standards of health and wellness.

Optimal health and wellness ought be measured with adjectives like *energetic, vibrant, ptimistic, relaxed, clear-headed, limber, agile, strong, peaceful*, and *fulfilled*. If this seems unrealistic or impossible, take a moment to examine how you feel right at this moment. You might find yourself experiencing symptoms such as tight muscles, sinus congestion, fatigue, or gastric discomfort that you might not even have been aware of, or that you might even consider "normal" because you usually feel that way. Now consider how frequently a symptom must be present to get your attention or even to act on it. Imagine the strain on the body from putting off these messages, and the body's only choice is to turn up the volume to get you to notice.

If we define "normal" by comparing our experience to those around us, then these symptoms and conditions might indeed seem normal. If, however, we define "normal" as natural and unavoidable, then nothing could be further from the truth. With the influences of stress and aging, we tend to accept declines in health as normal. Although some deterioration is inevitable, many of our debilitating age-related conditions have more to do with chronic lifestyle neglect than they do with age itself.

Imagine a beautiful Victorian house built 150 years ago. If the families that inhabited it never maintained it—never cleaned, repaired, painted, etc.—it would likely need upgrade or be in total disrepair. If, on the other hand, that house had been kept up and regularly maintained, today it would be a beautiful, historic, even antique home that someone might pay top dollar to own. Certainly, there would be some signs of wear and age, but for a house that has been well maintained, this would contribute to the house's character.

Similarly, if at age twenty or so we begin to focus exclusively on our career and raising a family; working long hours; eating on the run; and not leaving time for exercise, meditation, rest, massage, or other self-care, by the time we are thirty-five or forty we will be suffering from two decades' worth of neglect.

We are generally concerned with our health only when symptoms become intolerable. In the face of such discomfort, we are often satisfied with symptom management even when the precipitating condition still exists. This would be like painting the wall of our Victorian home to cover cracks resulting from a compromised foundation.

By contrast, in Okinawa, Tibet, Russia, and other parts of the world where food and water are pure and clean, spirituality is emphasized, stress is minimized, and a more primitive lifestyle requires regular exercise in the form of walking (and sometimes carrying heavy loads), it is not uncommon for people to live past one hundred years of age while still enjoying vigorous health and vitality. In fact, many of these countries have never even heard of cancer, diabetes, or ADHD. By learning from the example set in these remote Eastern cultures, we can choose to maintain ourselves the way we might maintain a Victorian home and enjoy a vibrant quality of life—even into late adulthood.

THE INTEGRATED NATURE OF DISEASE

Just as illness, injury, and other maladies need not be a normal part of the natural aging process, they are also, barring some exceptions, neither random nor unavoidable. While predisposition to illness may be encoded onto our DNA, it takes environmental stressors in the form of toxins, strain, and trauma to bring it out. Let's explore this concept by examining a common condition often thought of as genetic: allergies.

By definition, an allergy is a false autoimmune response. This means we came into contact with (or ingested) something harmless like grass, pollen, or animal dander, and our immune system mistook it for something dangerous like a virus or toxin. Our body goes to work to expel it by sneezing, creating a fever, creating excess mucus, coughing, and so on. In short, with allergies, as with all autoimmune conditions, the body attacks itself without good cause (like burning off a virus or expelling bacteria).

In the United States, most people suffering from allergies see an allergist, who treats them with inhalers, injections, and pills. Ironically, most of these people continue seeing these same allergists and taking these same treatments throughout their lives without any improvement in their health.

By contrast, there is a strong correlation between diet, lifestyle change, and relief from the symptoms of allergies. When the body's immune system functions optimally (from proper nutrition, hydration, rest, etc.), it no longer misidentifies benign objects as harmful, yet we seem to have accepted symptom management or decreased suffering as acceptable instead of insisting on a cure. Unfortunately, we share responsibility with the health-care community for this situation.

By accepting the status quo and not assuming responsibility for our own health management, we have enabled health-care providers to fill a role by medicating away our symptoms. We have given them responsibility for making us *feel* well instead of having them educate us and teach us to be self-reliant. Understanding this, however, we have the opportunity to accept responsibility for our own health care and maintenance. We can educate ourselves about prevention, integrated treatments, and holistic wellness and insist that our health-care providers focus more on promoting optimal wellness and illness prevention instead of managing our symptoms and keeping us ill.

UNDERSTANDING THE ROLE OF STRESS

By design, human beings need a certain type and amount of stress. Although an in-depth discussion of human stress response and its benefits are beyond the scope of this book, suffice it to say that human beings were designed for intervals of high-intensity stress with intermittent intervals of recovery and relaxation. For example, a life of farming, prayer, or craftsmanship might be periodically interrupted by an invading army, a hunt for food, or the need to run from a dangerous animal.

When exposed to this intermittent, high-intensity stress, our heart rate and blood pressure spike, our muscles get damaged from exertion, and we secrete hormones that interrupt digestion and elimination. Once the stressor is removed, we recover while resting, eating, and drinking. Our bodies' systems rebuild stronger and more capable than before. In fact, proper exercise design is based on this very model—periods of intense work followed by periods of rest, recovery, hydration, and good food.

Unfortunately, this lifestyle proves elusive in modern American culture. Instead of short periods of high-intensity stress, most people live under sustained, low-level (not life-threatening) stress such as work, money, and family pressure. Although these stressors are not life threatening, our bodies and minds respond as if they were. Living with this constant stress response (even at a low intensity) inhibits our ability to recover and taxes our immune system, preventing it from ever functioning optimally.

Add to this phenomenon the immune system's need to protect us from chemicals, hormones, and antibiotics in our food; the strain of dehydration; and pollutants such as cigarette smoke and engine exhaust in our air and water, and the stage is set for autoimmune-based chronic illness (allergies, lupus, asthma, etc.). By adjusting our lifestyles to better manage the physical and emotional stressors in our lives, and allowing for greater rest and recovery, we can dramatically limit, if not entirely eliminate, autoimmune conditions and their chronic threat to our quality of life.

LIFESTYLE VERSUS GENETICS

Many chronic ailments are considered "genetic" and thus unavoidable. Illnesses do reoccur within families, as you can probably attest to after a quick scan of your family tree. Genetics play an undeniable role in our health-related tendencies, both strengths and weaknesses. We are not, however, bound by genetic predetermination. We can inherit various threats to our well-being from our families through a combination of learned lifestyles, behaviors and habits, and latent predispositions. The good news is that we can avoid many these hazards by learning to better manage our lifestyle.

Some people are born with conditions like type 1 diabetes or multiple sclerosis. In these cases, the condition was predetermined via genetics, so the only way to mitigate the disease's symptoms is through lifestyle. It's more typical, however, to have greater volition in preventing disease. In most cases, our illnesses and conditions are entirely avoidable and are entirely reversible.

We learn our behaviors, habits, and coping skills from our families. If, for example, our parents tend to eat poorly and not exercise, we will grow up knowing this as normal, not always realizing healthier ways to eat and live. Ultimately, our dietary and lifestyle choices might set us up for type 2 diabetes just as our parents' choices contributed to their developing the same illness. Similarly, emotional distress such as depression likely has more to do with how we learned to cope with our difficulties (from watching our families) than with losing some genetic lottery.

What genetics do is outline our predispositions or tendencies—not necessarily our fate. If, for example, people in your family tend to store excess body fat in their bellies, or in their hips and thighs, you will likely store excess body fat in the same areas. This does not mean, however, that you must store excess body fat at all. Even if you have a genetically slow metabolism that makes it difficult for you to lose weight, you can, through more optimal channels such as proper diet and exercise programs, maintain a healthy weight throughout your life. Adhering to a proper diet and fitness program need not be difficult, but it does require some education. Not all diets and/or fitness programs are created equal. It might be worth consulting experts in these fields before making lifestyle changes.

Genetics will determine which ailments you might develop if you neglect your health (allergies, lupus, asthma, etc.), but, in most cases, lifestyle decisions will determine whether or not you get sick at all.

THE MODERN MEDICAL PARADIGM

Modern medical science has accomplished amazing feats. Where people once died in their teens and twenties due to acute infections and illnesses, influenza, and cuts/abrasions, we now enjoy long lives in which these acute infections seldom develop into more than minor inconveniences. Thanks to advances in surgical procedures, we can walk with prosthetic legs, survive major organ dysfunction with artificial heart valves, or overcome disease and injury with organ transplants. What's more, most bone, joint, and muscle injuries can be corrected in such a way that we can continue our lives without restricting ourselves in sports or other enjoyable activities.

Unfortunately, despite our ever-increasing knowledge and ability, we, as a culture, continue to get sicker and sicker. In the next two decades, new cancer cases worldwide are expected to rise from 8.2 million to 13 million.

We may attribute this staggering rate of cancer growth to longer life spans, but this may be only part of the picture. Since young people, as well as old, suffer from cancer and other physical/mental illness such as obesity, we might look outside the United States to understand this epidemic. Evidence there negates longevity as the primary factor, since people in other parts of the world often live longer than the average American while enjoying considerably better health and vitality. One conclusion is that a fundamental flaw in modern American health may have more to do with our paradigm of health and how we have learned to address illness.

The first of two primary limitations in our current health-care system has to do with the culture we have created. Between our high-powered careers and our family responsibilities, our lives have become so demanding that we find ourselves unable to take time for health maintenance practices like meditation, healthful eating, massage, or regular exercise, let alone rest and recovery when we do get sick. Instead, when we fall ill, we take medicines to treat our symptoms, allowing us to continue working, taking the kids to karate, and cooking dinner. We overlook the condition(s) damaging our bodies and taxing our immune systems because we feel well enough to do these things.

Instead of adjusting our lifestyles to accommodate (or prevent) illness, we adjust the illness to accommodate our lifestyles. Case in point, there used to be a condition called "adult onset diabetes." With the prominence of fast, convenient junk food and high-tech, sedentary lifestyles, more and more children began developing adult onset diabetes. We did not address the social conditions creating this phenomenon and instead renamed the disease type 2 diabetes so as not to discriminate against the millions of youths who have developed the condition.

The second concern with our current health-care system is that the business of medicine needs people to be sick. No gains are made by the established mainstream health-care industry when we are well. Physicians and pharmaceutical companies only make money when we are sick or believe ourselves to be unwell. The powerful forces that influence our perceptions of health and wellness are not fully considered, so much so that we don't flinch when flooded with commercials on medications with horrific side effects.

In ancient China, families used to pay their physician a monthly retainer to keep them well. In turn, the doctor designed the family's diet, exercise regime, meditation schedule, herbal supplements, and so on. If a member of the family did take ill, the doctor paid the family the monthly retainer until the person was well again. The doctor profited only if his patients were healthy. In fact, he lost money when their health suffered.

This is far from the case in the United States, with a business model in health care that does not reward prevention and health maintenance. In this country we may do more to keep our cars running well than our bodies. Just as regular oil changes, tire rotations, and tune-ups are necessary components in avoiding expensive car repairs, nutrition, hydration, exercise, and therapy must be necessary components in avoiding expensive and life-threatening disease. And just as fixing your car (brakes, transmission, etc.) when it needs repair is more important than covering the problem so you become less aware of it, creating health and wellness must become more important than simply managing illness so that we are less aware of it.

In order to facilitate change, we must change our mindset. We must no longer tolerate a medical business model that requires us to be ill for the industry to profit. Taking responsibility for our own wellness instead of expecting doctors to "fix" us is where we begin. If we take in the idea we aren't always broken, damaged, or afflicted, we might look at treatment as a process that begins at home.

Let's build a foundation in our medical and mental health-care paradigm that reflects the work of gestalt therapy, that a professional's job is not to "fix" our problems, but to be an expert facilitator of our own self-care. This is actually where health care began: in recognizing that the job of a doctor is to aid the body in its own natural healing process.

The good news is that a push for change seems to be growing. More people are turning to alternative healing methods like psychotherapy, nutrition, acupuncture/acupressure, herbal treatments, meditation, and exercise instead of traditional pharmaceuticals and surgeries. Managed care organizations are starting to cover alternative treatments and reimburse gym memberships in the name of prevention.

UNDERSTANDING THE IMPORTANCE OF SYMPTOMS

When we get sick, it's the symptoms of our illnesses that interfere with our lives. In the absence of these symptoms, we can continue to live and work with everything from a cold to cancer. Accordingly, most medications are designed to combat symptoms of illness—not to cure illness. Although the symptoms of illness can make it difficult or even impossible to function in our daily lives, our symptoms have two very important functions.

First, our bodies combat illness with symptoms. A fever, for example, is the body's way of creating an environment where bacteria cannot live, much the same way pasteurizing (heating) milk or boiling water kills the bacteria. In emotional struggles, too, symptoms are important. Thanks to the feedback we receive from our bodies, we know how we feel and what we might need in order to feel better.

Depression, anxiety, anger, and sadness are all accompanied by sensations or symptoms that let us know how we feel and what we need.

Although this concept might seem foreign, if we can learn to listen to our body's messages, we might gain insights into what we need and find ourselves able to make the adjustments that will help us grow and progress through a given struggle.

When our bellies grumble, the body is telling us we need food. If we pause and connect with our bellies (through images in our mind's eye) without distraction, we will likely see different foods like chicken, steak, pineapple, or salad. Often our bodies tell us what foods we want in order to address existing nutritional deficiencies. It is not uncommon for people with Crohn's disease (a digestive disorder) to crave cultured foods like yogurt, kimchi, and sauerkraut because the cultures in these foods aid in digestion.

Along these same lines, learning to listen to our bodies is often an important component of therapy, because doing so helps us better understand our reactions to other people, places, and situations. If we can listen to our anxiety or our depression, we might find that we also experience physical sensations in our bodies. Like when we are hungry, if we can connect with these messages from the body, we will likely learn what we need (i.e., safety, love, acceptance, challenge, etc.). If we medicate our symptoms away to gain the capacity to function better in certain areas, we run the risk of missing the opportunity to interpret this vital data, which is the key to feeling better or healing.

Second, simple as it might seem, our symptoms let us know that we are unwell so that we will slow our lives down and spend some time attending to our health. Medication can produce relief from symptoms that might give us a false sense of health or wellness. This false sense of wellness can be dangerous, because if the virus, bacteria, or emotional disturbance that created our symptoms still exists despite the absence of symptoms due to medication, we might not give ourselves the rest, nutrition, therapy, or other treatment we might need to overcome the illness. If we take painkillers for a broken arm, for example, in the absence of pain (the symptom), we might try to use the arm again, worsening the damage that has already been done.

PREVENTION

An ounce of prevention truly is worth a pound of the cure, and at no time has this been more true than today. Most people don't realize that taking an antibiotic can drastically reduce the good flora in our intestine that protects us from harmful bacteria, for up to a year. Or consider sleep problems and the millions of Americans who have become dependent on sleep medications because they didn't deal with their anxiety soon enough.

As described earlier, our current health-care system requires us to become ill in order for doctors, insurance companies, and pharmaceutical companies to prosper. Even therapy, when subsidized by health-care organizations, cannot be accessed unless a significant medical illness is diagnosed. Consequently, we learn to minimize problems unless they become too severe to ignore.

Rather than becoming complacent about our health, relying on innovations in medicine to keep us well, it's imperative we become more proactive and do it starting today. Health maintenance can become part of our lifestyle, which in the long run can help us save time and money, with fewer sick days and greater productivity. In spite of the cost of yoga, massage, organic foods, or a gym membership, they are just a fraction of what a year spent fighting cancer will cost.

Just as a small, periodic monetary investment in your car, such as an oil change, can help you avoid costly auto repairs, a similar commitment to maintaining your health and vitality can save you time and money on medications, frequent doctor visits, and even hospitalizations. Organic food is often more expensive than conventionally grown foods, but organic foods have also been correlated with a significant decrease in allergies, asthma, ADHD, depression, and other maladies. The extra money spent on higher-quality foods pales in comparison to the cost of treating any one (let alone a combination of) the aforementioned conditions, the cost of lower productivity due to compromised work performance, and money lost by taking time off from work due to illness.

Attention to health maintenance and illness prevention requires a paradigm shift. Those interested in experiencing optimum health and vitality must begin to focus on wholeness. Where our current medical paradigm breaks us down into small, specialized parts (therapists; podiatrists; allergists; proctologists; shoulder specialists; ear, nose, and throat specialists, etc.), the shift to wholeness implies that the whole is greater than the sum of its parts. Improved health means refraining from isolating problems by clustering symptoms and seeking out specialists. The body is an organism, with many interwoven systems that are influenced by countless factors, both internal and external.

Although a specialist might be appropriate when a particular condition or injury does arise, in terms of prevention, we can no more care only for the health of our left elbow over the rest our bodies than we can separate the physical from the mental and emotional. Remember that everything is connected with everything else, so realize the systemic nature of issues for optimum prevention and intervention.

DEFINING THE WHOLENESS CENTER

As the public's interest in prevention and holistic wellness grows, facilities providing integrated health solutions begin to emerge. Sometimes referred to as "wellness centers," "alternative health centers," "integrated wellness centers," or "wholeness centers," these facilities strive to offer the health-care consumer natural, nonpharmaceutical, nonsurgical treatment and prevention options that integrate mental, physical, and sometimes spiritual health.

In researching wholeness centers, one might find any combination of psychotherapists, massage therapists, yoga instructors, Rolfers, personal trainers, Feldenkrais instructors, nutritionists, apothecaries, naturopathic doctors, chiropractors, acupuncturists, meditation teachers, and clergy. Occasionally, an assortment of the aforementioned professionals will keep offices in the same building or strip mall. Sometimes they will not occupy the same physical space but will work together as a wellness network nonetheless.

Choosing a wholeness center can be a challenging proposition. Although many such centers legitimately strive to help people improve their health practices and related education by staffing themselves with educated, licensed/certified professionals who are committed to continuing education and excellence in practice, some centers are simply exercise studios, massage parlors, or diet centers with names that might prove misleading.

There may be nothing inherently wrong with these facilities, but if they do not attend to mental/emotional health, nutrition, disease prevention/treatment, and spirituality, as well as physical health, then they are limited in helping their clients move toward wholeness. Other centers may indeed address mental, physical, and spiritual wellness but do so through different disciplines.

BECOMING AN INVOLVED WELLNESS CONSUMER

Should you choose a wholeness center offering yoga, psychotherapy, and herbal medicine, or one that combines counseling, physical fitness, and nutrition? There is more than one road to our desired destination, and any choice will likely yield valuable results. However, getting a feel for the care coordinator can help you appreciate how structured the facility is, matching your need for direction. In becoming more self-reliant and assuming responsibility for our own wellness, we first identify specific needs and preferences and then find the facility that best accommodates our individual situation. For routine maintenance, a less structured facility may work, but for more pinpointed and acute issues, something more guided may be helpful.

Because wholeness centers are still uncommon, you might find it difficult to locate any such facility to accommodate all your specific needs. Until a local center is established, you may need to design your own wellness "team," including a therapist, personal trainer, nutritionist, and massage therapist. Even if they practice independently, you, as their client, can empower them to communicate with one another in order to develop a complete, cohesive lifestyle plan on your behalf.

In researching wholeness centers (or assembling a wholeness team of your own), you must ensure the providers you choose are qualified. While certain professionals such as psychologists, registered dietitians, and naturopathic doctors must have specific degrees from accredited universities and state licenses to practice legally, other practitioners like personal trainers, nutritionists, and massage therapists might not need any formal credential to practice legally in your state.

If these professionals do possess credentials, understand that not all certifications are equivalent. Personal training credentials, for example, can range from passing an online examination after reading an article on the certifying organization's website to passing a battery of written and practical exams after an intensive six- to twelve-month study period. The educated consumer might benefit from researching specific credentials before hiring professionals to help manage his or her health.

So often, in buying a car, choosing investments, hiring a landscaper, or picking out furniture, we comparison shop, look for sales, and research consumer reports. We put energy into ensuring that we buy the right products for the best prices or choose the best investments for our finances. Yet we often ignore health matters until we become ill. Then we see any doctor that will accept our insurance, accept his or her diagnosis, and follow his or her subsequent medical advice without question.

If we can learn to maintain our wellness, especially before we take ill; integrate emotional, physical, nutritional, and spiritual practices in order to approach wholeness; and exercise the same judgment and scrutiny in employing health-care professionals as we do employing other professionals, we can pave the road to a long life of optimal health and vitality.

Interesting Facts

- By 2020, major depressive illness will be the leading cause of disability in the world for women and children.[1]
- Stigma erodes confidence that mental disorders are real, treatable health conditions.[2]
- The economic cost of untreated mental illness is more than $100 billion each year in the United States.[3]
- It's important to address an illness on both an emotional and physical level.[4]
- Optimism can improve physical health.[5]
- Psychology can help family and loved ones cope with the effects of a serious or life-threatening illness.[6]
- Psychology can help manage the side effects of medical treatments.[7]
- Studies have shown if the mind is in good shape, then the quality of life is better.[8]

12

ALTERNATIVE HEALTH CARE

The collective conscience and will of our profession is being tested as never before. Now is the time for us to have the courage for legendary work. —Dr. Caldwell B. Esselstyn Jr.

The path to wellness is less about one particular course and more about multiple roads, all leading you toward the same place. Along this path you will enlist the help of many people, both professionals and nonprofessionals. You will read books and articles. You may research on the Internet or attend lectures. You will take all the information you have obtained to consider what fits for you and what gets discarded. Because the path to wellness is about becoming more whole, integrating the different parts of yourself to be powerful, increase your vitality, and deepen your contact with others, you will sometimes steer toward less-traditional types of ideas to help you reach these goals.

In this chapter we will visit with some of the alternative approaches, which are named this way only because they are not considered traditional or standard from a perspective that is fading. In fact, these approaches and ancillary services are becoming increasingly common in a global society where consumers are more guided by natural pathways toward wellness. Some of these approaches may seem as though they are more germane to physical health, so remember that we are interconnected between physical, psychological, and spiritual wellness, the combinations of which are unique to each person. If we improve one area, the other areas will likely be impacted.

Holistic, naturopathic, or homeopathic approaches to wellness can be transformative, but also confusing for the newcomer. For someone with cancer who hasn't had success with traditional medicine such as chemotherapy or radiation therapy, the prospect of an alternative wellness model may be appealing. For others, especially those not living in a more contemporary community, alternative health practices may be lesser known and even feared as mythical. For the vast majority of us, alternative health care may range from chiropractors to acupuncture with much in between.

For those who haven't yet considered alternative health care, we may be old-fashioned in our views, skeptical of its efficacy, or loyal to mainstream medicine. We must admit that our heavy reliance on pharmaceuticals in this country has helped to steer our beliefs, following the paradigm that an advanced society with successes in genetic engineering can help us to overcome anything that ails us. While there may be truth to this statement, it's also possible to go too far in the direction of overreliance.

For the millions who rush to their primary care physician with a cold, seeking antibiotics, this couldn't be any more true. Nobody likes to suffer, and we have come to expect that treatments are easily accessible and harmless. This, however, is not always the case. Many who are prescribed antibiotics, who are suffering from a cold (virus), will not be helped and in fact may be harmed.

According to Dr. Joel Fuhrman, the author of *Super Immunity* and *Disease-Proof Your Child*,[1] taking one dose of antibiotics can reduce the good flora in our intestine for up to a year. The loss of good flora can reduce our resistance to bacteria and lead to increased vulnerability to illness. The same author also noted that the more antibiotics we take, the greater the risk of breast cancer for women, which is an issue receiving more attention of late.

If you ask T. Colin Campbell, the author of *The China Study*, which is the largest piece of research ever conducted on nutrition, there is a definitive link between casein and cancer. Casein is a protein found in milk and red meat. Because of the influences of the dairy and agriculture industries, we have been persuaded that health is the opposite of what these findings support.

Enter this next section with an open mind, allowing yourself to recognize beliefs that have been internalized around health. Some of these approaches may seem commonsensical or even mystical, yet their following seems to grow each day.

NUTRITION

Our eating habits are largely underestimated as a cause of and contributor to all types of dis-ease. We tend to view healthy eating as common sense, making us more reluctant to seek out professional support. Adding to our resistance is the ever-changing research that tells us something is good for us one day and then bad for us the next.

Triglycerides used to be the culprit for people who ate fatty food. Mainstream diets such as Atkins recently blamed carbohydrates . Salt has been a long-standing no-no that was linked with high blood pressure. If we search any of these items, we can find balanced research that suggests worse problems to look out for.

The reality is that nutrition is a complex science, and even those with good eating patterns will benefit from working with a trained expert in the field. As many commonalities as we have as corporal beings, we also have distinct differences. Consider a person with ulcerative colitis who believes that raw vegetables (an important element of health for humans) feel sadistic when pushed on them, or a person who never smokes, eats only unprocessed foods, and still is stricken with cancer.

You will want to be careful, though, because there are many different types of nutritional counselors, including dietitians, certificate holders of various paradigms, nutritional consultants, and others. It's not easy to figure out who has the right training to help. A simple way to rule out potential professionals is to ask them about the information in this chapter. A general overview of the distinctions within this field is as follows.

- Diplomat of the American Clinical Board of Nutrition: All professionals at the doctorate level who qualify can sit for the two-part exam. Diplomats are most commonly chiropractors and often work in clinics and private practice. They are certified by the American Clinical Board of Nutrition.
- Registered dietitian: RDs have a minimum of a bachelor's degree, trained as generalists in both typical and medical food-related issues. Most dietitians, after getting their required number of training

hours, work in medical settings such as hospitals, clinics, and nursing homes. RDs are credentialed by the Commission on Dietetic Registration of the Academy of Nutrition and Dietetics.

- Certified nutrition specialist: Must have a master's degree or a doctorate in nutrition or a doctorate in clinical health care from a regionally accredited university as well as one thousand hours of supervised experience. They must pass a four-hour board exam on medical nutrition therapy, then go on to work in clinics, private practices, or community settings. They are credentialed by the Certification Board for Nutrition Specialists.

- Certified clinical nutritionist: Requires a bachelor's degree, a nine-hundred-hour internship, and fifty-six hours of online, postgraduate study in clinical nutrition or a master's degree in human nutrition. Their training may be more unique, approaching clients based on individual issues, with work done in clinics and private practice. They are credentialed by the Clinical Nutrition Certification Board.

- Certified nutritionist: Credential involves completing a six-course distance-learning program and passing a proctored exam, which is offered through American Health Science University.

- Holistic nutritionist: Must have a degree from an approved holistic nutrition program and five hundred hours of professional experience in the field. Practitioners don't necessarily follow the government food pyramid guidelines. They do not practice medical nutrition therapy or diagnose disease. They are certified by the Holistic Nutrition Credentialing Board, a division of the National Association of Nutrition Professionals.

- Certified health coach: More schools and programs are offering this track than ever before. The Institute for Integrative Nutrition, one of the larger schools to certify health coaches, offers a yearlong online course that covers one hundred dietary theories, ranging from the paleo diet to raw foods. Health coaches set goals with, support, and educate clients toward achieving personal wellness goals.

- Certified nutrition consultant: Must have a high school diploma or GED and complete a series of eleven open-book tests, which candidates have a maximum of five years to finish. They are credentialed by the American Association of Nutrition Consultants, a group that opposes licensure and registration.

It is important to consider whether a nutritional advocate knows about genetically modified organisms (GMOs). Most of the country is just starting to learn about GMOs and their growing threat to both the food industry and our health. The simple but powerful facts to consider: The same company that brought us DDT, Agent Orange, and Roundup now also owns nearly 70 percent of the world's seed supply. And what are they doing with our seeds? They are inserting pesticides into the genes of these seeds to create a different plant species, one that has proven harmful to farmers and to people who ingest them.

It's a terrible cycle this company (Monsanto) has created. They develop crops like Roundup Ready soybeans and supply the feed to our livestock, which in turn get sick, requiring antibiotics. Now we are eating meat that has added steroids (to increase the amount of meat and their revenue) and antibiotics, making us more resistant to illness because the medicines we take don't work as well and cause the germs to morph into new strands. We are in a downward spiral where heirloom seeds are harder to find because the spread of these modified seeds through the air contaminates the pure ones. It's a vicious cycle that goes well beyond what I've described, and the concerned reader will want to get involved.

If looking into the decline of our food industry is too much, let's stay with finding the right nutritional consultant for now. In addition to wanting them knowledgeable about GMOs, we need somebody who appreciates the biological and chemical factors of food. For instance, they need to know that phytochemicals are elements that strengthen and support normal immune function. They are not vitamins or minerals.

Nutrition advocates will also need to know that antioxidants are vitamins, minerals, and phytochemicals that remove the "free radicals" and control free radical production; they include the carotene family (lycopene, beta-carotene, lutein, and zeaxanthin). Other compounds that promote the healing properties of cells include alpha-lipoic acid, flavonoids, bioflavonoids, polyphenols, phenolic acids, quercetin, rutin, anthocyanins, proanthocyanins, allium compounds, allylsulfides, glucosinolates, isothiocyanates, lignans, and pectins. Antioxidants are the natural enemy of free radicals, which are unpaired, highly chemically reactive electrons. These unstable molecules are destructive when they come into contact with our cells.

An excess of free radicals causes inflammation and promotes aging. Inflammation is often the beginning of the disease process. Free radicals eat up waste in the body, which can aid in the prevention of cancer, but when their numbers increase (due to too few antioxidants), they move outside their specified area and start destroying healthy cells. Apoptosis is the process of fighting cancerous or precancerous cells before they can harm the body. These are all facts your nutritional consultant should know.

You may also ask your nutritional expert if they appreciate the potential link between gluten (from wheat) and the rise of ADHD. Some believe that our year-round exposure to gluten, which was once available only during certain points of the growing season, is causing us harm. There is a valid argument for this with the rise of allergies, asthma, ADHD, autism, and other childhood ailments, but there are numerous other possibilities for who is to blame.

We could point the finger at the thousands of harmful environmental toxins, many of which come from plastics. We could look into the steroids and antibiotics being given to our livestock, or even the use of pesticides and GMOs as a likely source of our declining health. The reality is that many if not all of these factors plus more make up the expanding links in a chain that is choking off our attempts to be healthy.

With the alarming rise in cancer being predicted (57 percent in the next twenty years worldwide), we can no longer be complacent about our health. To alleviate suffering, whether it's physiological or psychological, we need to move away from a single point of focus into a much broader perspective of health and wellness. The multiple factors that influence health require all the providers in different fields to pool their knowledge to shield us from the growing number of threats to our health.

The question of vitamins won't be covered here; suffice it to say that controversy exists over their efficacy. Those who can't or won't get their vitamins and minerals from food are left with the temptation to substitute with supplements. For people who eat unprocessed foods and a high concentration of both raw and cooked vegetables and fruits, the need for vitamins may not be strong. While there may not be any harm in adding vitamins to your diet, the goal is always to get these elements met as naturally as possible. If you do take a vitamin, consider whether it has toxic ingredients, as many do, whether it is derived from food without artificial substitutes, or whether it is overengineered.

Even for those who believe they are doing all the right things, there is yet another concern to be mindful of. Because of soil depletion, even an adequate amount of fruits and vegetables every day may not be meeting our dietary needs. If the soil is lacking in important elements such as magnesium, phosphorus, nitrogen, calcium, potassium, zinc, copper, manganese, boron, iron, and the hundreds of others, then your apple may be only a third of what it used to be.

The main message is to avoid complacency about your nutrition. Not only is nutrition important for your health and longevity, but the problems in our food industry are impacting the wellness of our planet. If China is refusing U.S. exports of corn and Russia has banned the use of GMOs in their country, why is the United States so **complacent about the issue**?

Here are some great resources to consider about your health and the sociopolitical influences that may be affecting you without your realizing it.

Resource List

Movies

- *Genetic Roulette*
- *Food Matters*
- *Forks over Knives*
- *Hungry for Change*
- *Food Inc.*
- *Farmageddon*
- *The World According to Monsanto*
- *Supersize Me*
- *Got the Facts on Milk?*
- *Fat, Sick and Nearly Dead*

Books

- *Super Immunity*
- *Disease-Proof Your Child*
- *Seeds of Deception*
- *The China Study*
- *Food Politics*
- *Appetite for Profit*
- *The End of Food*

- *Fast Food Nation*
- *Sweetness and Power*
- *The Starch Solution*
- *The Omnivore's Dilemma*

While much of this section is devoted to nutrition as it relates to our physical health, there is also a direct correlation (as well as indirect through physical health) to our psychological well-being. Research is increasing on the role of nutrition and how it ties into emotional wellness, gaining steam every day. A fifteen-day online anxiety summit concluded in June 2014, for instance, the sole purpose of which was to link nutrition and anxiety. A quick scan of the Internet will show hundreds of links to other maladies such as depression which can also be linked to nutrition, not simply because the body is rundown and lethargic, but also because of the impact on neurotransmitters and other direct correlates to emotional well-being.

When researching therapists or other helping professionals, selecting one that has either a knowledge of nutrition or at minimum an apprecia-tion of the role of healthy eating should influence your decision. As our growing awareness helps us appreciate the interconnectivity between our physical and emotional health, it's that much more important to have a professional who can help us to link all these areas, even if they aren't the one to address it themselves.

YOGA

Yoga is an ancient form of exercise originating in India around five thousand years ago. An Indian sage, Patanjali, has been credited with bringing the oral tradition of yoga into his classical work, *The Yoga Sutras*. In this collection Patanjali provides a philosophical guide to the practice of yoga.

In America, we think of yoga as an exercise program that will make us strong and flexible. Yoga can do this, but the philosophy of yoga focuses as much on our spiritual development. It is believed that working the body through a series of movements in concert with changing the way we breathe will connect us to our spirit and inner wisdom.

Whatever your reasons are for doing yoga, everyone can benefit on a physical, emotional, and spiritual level. In most classes all of these aspects may be incorporated, but it's often left up to the student as to which are paramount. Most classes begin with centering and breath work followed by warm-ups, postures, and relaxation/meditation at the end. You do not have to be flexible or strong; just have an open mind and an open heart. We think of yoga as one of life's journeys, and we hope that it becomes a part of your everyday life as it has for us.

Namaste is a term often heard in yoga centers, representing the belief that a divine spark within each of us is located in the heart chakra. The gesture is an acknowledgment of the soul in one by the soul in another. *Nama* means "bow," *as* means "I," and *te* means "you." Therefore, *namaste* literally means "bow me you" or "I bow to you."

Keep in mind there are many types of yoga, so finding the right application is important. Oftentimes people get discouraged before or shortly after starting. Some believe they aren't flexible or patient enough, or they don't think they can get their minds to slow down well enough to use this medium. For those who stick with it, finding the right level of class, type of yoga, and environment that suits them, yoga can be enriching on several levels.

With a growing trend in "mindfulness," a broad spectrum of therapies that now emphasize living in the moment, we may appreciate even more what yoga has been advocating for many years. If we can set our intentions, clear our minds, and allow our bodies time to heal, we will feel more whole and have greater energy. For anybody engaged in therapy, yoga is a wonderful complement to wellness.

Yoga can complement the therapy process in many ways. Those who are anxious may learn how to slow down and respect their bodies. Those who are depressed can generate energy from becoming more fully integrated, and for those who are suffering from compulsions of any kind (i.e., addictions or dependencies), it's a way of getting more in touch with drives that aren't linked to our thinking.

MASSAGE

There are many forms of massage therapy, including Swedish, deep tissue, Shiatsu, and Thai, among many others. The benefits include an increase in circulation, a decrease in the stress hormone cortisol, a lowering of blood pressure, a reduction in the buildup of lactic acid, and an overall sense of relaxation and mind clearing, among others.

Swedish massage is the most common type in the United States. Massage therapists, most of whom require licenses in the majority of states, use long, smooth strokes, kneading, and circular movements on superficial layers of muscle, using massage lotion or oil. This is different from deep tissue massage, which targets deeper layers of muscle and connective tissue. Deep tissue massage is used for chronically tight or painful muscles, repetitive strain, postural problems, or recovery from injury. People often feel sore for one to two days after deep tissue massage.

Reflexology is sometimes called foot massage, involving pressure to certain points on the foot that correspond to organs and systems in the body. Sports massage is designed for those who are involved in physical activity. The focus isn't on relaxation but on preventing and treating injury and enhancing athletic performance.

Shiatsu is a form of Japanese bodywork that uses localized finger pressure in a rhythmic sequence on acupuncture meridians. Each point is held for two to eight seconds to improve the flow of energy and help the body regain balance. Thai also intends to align the body's energies by using gentle pressure on specific points. Thai massage also includes compressions and stretches.

Other types of massage use stimulation other than oil or target specific populations. Aromatherapy, for instance, uses scented plant oils that are relaxing, energizing, stress reducing, and balancing, such as lavender. Hot stone massage involves the placement of warm or hot stones on certain points to warm and loosen tight muscles and balance energy centers in the body.

Specific to a population is pregnancy massage, which requires specialized training before one can be approved. These practitioners know the proper way to position and support the woman's body during the massage and how to modify techniques. Back massage in contrast is for anybody who has specific back and neck issues, which is the chief complaint of people seeing a massage therapist.

One caution about massage is that the body is producing tension for a reason, so while massage may feel good, we are leaving our healing up to someone else. If we don't learn from what our body is telling us through its signaling, we may be left repeating similar patterns, looking outward instead of inward for healing.

In addition to being a phenomenal preventive medicine for all types of physical and psychological ailments, massage can be a tremendous addendum to any path to wellness. The experience of being touched in a gentle and caring manner alone is critical, let alone the help it provides with raising our awareness of where we store energy. Injuries and illnesses nearly always have an element of neglected tension in our bodies, which raises the potential for problems.

For people who have suffered some type of abuse as a child, massage may seem scary or unpleasant. The prospect of having a stranger put their hands on you may even feel injurious. Keep in mind that experienced massage therapists can work with you to help you work through this discomfort, in a way that traditional therapy may not.

A theoretical approach called the Synergy Method, created by Ilana Rubenfeld, even combines the idea of touch and therapy. While it may not be easy to find a practitioner who uses this, it can be a life-changing experience when done by an experienced therapist.

REIKI

Reiki is a Japanese technique for stress reduction and relaxation that also promotes healing. The word *Reiki* is made of two Japanese words—*Rei*, which means "God's wisdom or the higher power," and *Ki*, which is "life force energy." So Reiki is actually "spiritually guided life force energy." It's administered by "laying on hands" and is based on the idea that an unseen "life force energy" flows through us, proving where there's life but also where there are blocks to healthy living. If our "life force energy" is low, then we are more likely to get sick or feel stress, and if it is high, we are more capable of happiness and health.

Reiki practitioners and masters tune in to the body's energy, sensing where flows are interrupted or needing restoration. While it is difficult to prove scientifically what the benefits are, those who enjoy this experience cite everything from the value of gentle touch to much deeper spiritual awakenings. It pulls from the belief that the body and mind can heal themselves and that disturbances in the individual's aura or chi, or life force that surrounds the body, are responsible for emotional and physical dis-eases.

The Reiki practitioner works within the aura field and the body's seven chakra points to rebalance the individual's life force. Each treatment is different, and each person experiences something different, as does the practitioner. Both the individual and the practitioner may feel things such as cool or warm temperatures; tingling; a sense of touch, images, and/or colors in their minds; and a myriad of other sensations. Reiki is rooted in intention, and the practitioner's energy exchange with the individual varies from person to person.

Reiki is ideal for people who, for physical limitations, can't receive a massage. It is also an excellent therapy complement for those who have experienced severe trauma and emotional distress. As with massage therapy, emotional release is common with Reiki, as it can bring many intense feelings to the surface as the body's life force is healed.

Other, even more esoteric means of achieving health and healing come from energy/spiritual work, such as angel card and tarot card readings, tai chi, meditation, and much more. All the approaches are too numerous to mention, but they share common elements of wanting healing to come from within instead of being externally applied. The goal for these practices is to empower and reduce reliance on traditional forms of helping that benefit from your dependence and not your independence.

Intuitive or spiritual counseling encourages enhanced perspective through the application of highly tuned intuition on the part of a spiritual counseling practitioner. By "tuning in" to the energy field and vibration of the client, they can enhance the attunement of the client. Most people using alternatives come with an acceptance of spirit or a soul, God, angels, spirit guides, or something intangible that we cannot see or measure but that is available to each of us as a powerful ally in our struggles as human beings.

Not all therapists pay attention to energy the way a Reiki master will; however, many of the more contemporary practitioners using less strategic approaches will incorporate energy work into their practice in some form. Simply paying attention to the body, recognizing one's relationship with the surrounding world, or learning how to draw energy from one's connection with the environment are ways of attending to this invisible force, so vital in moving toward wellness.

Interesting Facts

- The 2007 National Health Interview Survey found that 19.2 percent of American adults and 4.3 percent of children aged 17 and younger had used at least one complementary alternative medicine (CAM) mind-body therapy in the year prior to the survey.[2]
- Many studies document that psychological stress is linked to a variety of health problems, such as increased heart disease, compromised immune system functioning, and premature cellular and cognitive aging. Some evidence suggests that mind-body therapies could reduce psychological stress.[3]
- Pain sufferers often seek relief though CAM therapies, including mind-body modalities. A review of the evidence on various mind-body therapies to help treat certain neurological diseases involving pain found some evidence for positive effects from some therapies—including biofeedback for migraine headache, yoga for fatigue from multiple sclerosis, and relaxation therapy as a part of comprehensive programs to help control epileptic seizures.[4]
- In a study of sixty breast cancer survivors, women who used hypnosis reduced the number and severity of hot flashes and also reported improvements in mood and sleep.[5]
- A small preliminary trial suggests that Zen meditation may help prevent and/or reduce the cognitive decline of normal aging.[6]
- A study of sixty-three people with rheumatoid arthritis found that Mindfulness Based Stress Reduction helped to improve quality of life and reduce psychological distress.[7]
- A study of 298 college students found that Transcendental Meditation helped students reduce stress and improve coping strategies.[8]
- In a study of fifty women, regular practice of yoga benefited mood and physiological response to stress.[9]
- People with fibromyalgia may benefit from practicing tai chi, according to a study of sixty-six people. Study participants who practiced tai chi had a significantly greater decrease in total score on the Fibromyalgia Impact Questionnaire. In addition, the tai chi group demonstrated greater improvement in sleep quality, mood, and quality of life.[10]
- Tai chi may also be a safe alternative to conventional exercise for maintaining bone mineral density in postmenopausal women, thus

helping to prevent or slow osteoporosis, increase musculoskeletal strength, and improve balance.[11]

13

OTHER CONSIDERATIONS

You can sift through the following list in order to avoid some of the common pitfalls that clients often encounter in therapy. The list is by no means exhaustive, but it should be enough to help you prepare for what lies ahead. Consider it a compilation from thousands of client experiences over twenty-five years, from the experience of multiple clinicians.

COMMON MISTAKES: BY THE CLIENT

- Missing appointments
- Being unprepared
- Leaving therapy at the door (assimilation)
- Lacking direction
- All thought, no action
- Leaving therapy when "symptoms" abate
- Not telling the therapist when your needs aren't getting met
- Lacking patience/rushing progress
- Keeping therapy private
- Self-deprecation

Missing Appointments

It is particularly important to be consistent with your scheduled sessions, especially at the start of therapy. Imagine pushing a large boulder up an incline—the momentum you generate from the initial expenditure of energy is more easily sustained than it is if you stop pushing and have to start again. Due to a natural resistance to change, or at least the reluctance you may experience regarding the very personal issues you bring to therapy, the temptation may be to take mental breaks.

If you feel inundated with the work of therapy, it is best to talk about this and perhaps schedule a break. The alternative is forgetting a session, coming late, or even milling around during a session that may leave you feeling unproductive. You want to get the most out of your time, but it's difficult to carve out a consistent hour each week. In particular for those who aren't good at self-care, a regular appointment may be the first challenge on your path to wellness.

Being Unprepared

Many people arrive at therapy knowing they aren't happy but unsure what to do about it. After all, if you knew what to do, you might not be coming to therapy. Rather than viewing the therapist as the expert who is going to fix you, it is important to reconceptualize therapy as a vehicle as opposed to a cure. How you navigate the vehicle, such as how quickly you travel and how willing you are to explore alternative courses, determines the degree of success. Therapy is more like a guided tour where you are an active participant, as opposed to an instruction manual.

With that said, it's important you arrive at sessions prepared to work. If you come in without anticipating what work you want to do, you may spend valuable time milling around. Your therapist may help you to determine in what direction you might want to head, but the greater your reliance on this navigator, the less self-determination you experience. The ultimate goal of therapy, after all, is greater self-sufficiency, so the sooner you start this in therapy, the closer you will be upon termination.

Leaving Therapy at the Door (Assimilation)

Therapy is a concentrated time of self-exploration. Over time, it should become a spark plug for your work as opposed to your sole method of personal growth. The work done during sessions is designed to enhance your awareness toward a greater understanding of "what is" in order to determine what might be.

If you spend time following your session assimilating what was discussed, you may likely find further insight gained during the session. What is said to you during the session by the therapist might not always register at that point due to the layers of self-protection we commonly employ. Contemplation postsession can help open doors that were only slightly ajar earlier.

If your only time of reflection is inside the therapy office, you will slow down your work and possibly get discouraged by a lack of progress. Making time for yourself outside of the therapy session means you are extrapolating what you are learning and reminding yourself that helping others means first being good to yourself.

LACKING DIRECTION

Not selecting clear, concise, attainable, or sometimes measurable goals can leave you meandering through therapy. This may be somewhat confusing, because goals can be looked at in a couple of ways. More contemporary therapists, particularly ones that employ a more pragmatic approach such as cognitive behavioral, will advocate for specific and concrete goal setting because it lets you assess success. Additionally, it helps you to strategize what steps you are going to take when you know your intended outcome. This is similar to driving toward a particular destination as opposed to a region, which allows for better course plotting.

Another way of looking at this is through the lens of transformational change. This type of change process pays greater attention to how you are getting somewhere than where you are headed. For instance, a young man comes to therapy complaining of panic attacks. He is insistent that the therapist provide him with strategies to "get rid of" the anxiety. He was rewarded by previous therapists who taught relaxation techniques that initially helped decrease the worry. Unfortunately, this young man relapsed into panic shortly following conclusion of his sessions with these therapists.

It is likely the reason for this relapse was that this young man didn't explore the underlying issues creating the anxiety. Fortunately, he found a therapist months later who challenged him on his desire for a quick fix. The therapist helped him to explore the way in which he was looking at and trying to address this complicated issue, as opposed to moving him quickly toward problem resolution.

All Thought, No Action

Experiments have been defined as the risk-taking or creative actions that clients take based on the insight they gain through the course of therapy. Experiments allow you to experience yourself doing something outside your usual realm of action. For instance, if you argue with your spouse by telling him or her everything he or she does wrong, then an experiment might be to pay attention only to the things you are doing.

If most of your experimentation comes outside the session, your growth will be exponentially increased. If you reserve your risk taking for the session alone and don't give much consideration to what risks you can take in your life, you may remain stuck.

It's understandable that therapy is a safe place to move outside your comfort zone, but eventually you want to expand your work outside the office.

Leaving Therapy When "Symptoms" Abate

It's common for people to discontinue therapy when they begin to feel better. After all, therapy is an investment of time, energy, and money that takes away from other important obligations in your life. Most people coming to therapy for the first time are satisfied with resolving their initial concerns rather than making a commitment to personal growth work, which isn't necessarily a mistake, but ought to be considered before ending.

The danger with leaving therapy prematurely is that you can feel better without addressing the underlying issues that may resurface. The act of simply unburdening oneself can lead to feeling better, but this should not be confused with significant change. A person can rebound into discomfort similar or related to what originally brought them to therapy, but the second time around may be more discouraging. The person can feel worse because he or she adds the disappointment of the perceived setback.

Not Telling the Therapist When Your Needs Aren't Getting Met

Therapists are far from perfect. Their efforts to help may inadvertently harm or cause discomfort. Even a therapist's actions intended to alleviate suffering may not be effective, and the only way a clinician can measure his or her approach is through client feedback. Willingness to share your thoughts and feelings about what is happening in therapy can prevent the rifts that sometimes lead to premature termination of therapy. Many therapists are receptive to hearing your experience, even if involves unhappiness they may have created, because it says to them you have trust in the relationship.

Lacking Patience/Rushing Progress

It can take a lifetime to develop the concerns that bring us to therapy, yet we often wish for immediate alleviation of discomfort. Therapy unfortunately does not create miraculous cures; instead, it involves hard work that invites strong resistance to change. If we push too hard or go too fast, we might invite deeper heel-digging that can slow down the growth process.

If you give in to the temptation of feeling better quickly, you will gravitate toward therapists who are symptom focused. While a new relaxation technique or assertiveness skill can be applied quickly, make certain you aren't overlooking more deeply rooted causes for what ails you. If you become impatient, the therapist may feel this, and a less experienced clinician may start to rush their work, which is a setup for failure.

Keeping Therapy Private

Many people elect not to even tell others they are in therapy because it's embarrassing, a sign of weakness, or you are too private. You may fear unwanted questions or inquiries into your business and feel unable to set appropriate limits. Perhaps it's because you don't trust those people in your life to keep the information confidential, so you go through the experience alone.

The unfortunate part of keeping therapy private is a lack of support during a time when your energy may be drained. It can also be helpful to have a support system that can witness your experiments and provide feedback, test-driving the work done inside of session. When you share something so personal as being in therapy, others tend to respond by opening up about themselves, improving intimacy.

Self-Deprecation

The more work you do in therapy, the more likely you are to find work worth doing. At first, it can seem like a never-ending abyss of issues, even discouraging to those who view the "work" as tiresome. Feeling as though we are beyond repair, or at least "really screwed up," is common for those who discover deeper work along their journey.

If you look at therapy as a place to come to terms with your dark side, realizing that our frailties and inequities make us interesting and unique, we can resist the temptation to label ourselves as worthless. Refusing to equate damaged with worthless will allow you to remain curious and open, instead of divesting energy into salvaging self-esteem.

COMMON MISTAKES: BY THE THERAPIST

- Too lenient about collecting fees
- Steering away from "hot topics"
- Too aloof or too chatty
- Taking sides (couples therapy)
- Giving too much advice
- Insufficient feedback
- Being too much of an "expert"
- Taking too much or too little responsibility
- Not recognizing our own "stuff"
- Not challenging or confronting complacency
- Not meeting clients where they are
- Not addressing the therapeutic relationship
- Ignoring issues of diversity (gender, sexuality, ethnicity, etc.)
- Poor boundaries (being your friend)

Too Lenient about Collecting Fees

Many therapists are attracted to the helping profession because they care about people. This often means not being as focused on the business aspect of their profession, such as collecting fees. This can lead to problems because clients, particularly those whose troubles are influenced by or directly related to financial distress, may inadvertently take advantage of their therapist's kindness. Consider the following scenario:

A client has been coming to therapy for several months, occasionally neglecting his co-pay. On one occasion, this client forgets to cancel his appointment, leading to an additional fee that raises his balance even higher. The therapist reminds the client of this at times but has difficulty being firm. The resentment builds on the part of the therapist but comes out indirectly, such as paying less attention during sessions or providing fewer openings for the client to schedule appointments. This is not done intentionally but is due to feelings that have not been expressed. Now the potential for sabotage to the therapy exists, all because of money.

Steering Away from "Hot Topics"

Therapists are human and, because of this, they have similar responses to human suffering. When clients are nearing areas of their work that elicit strong feelings in a therapist, there may be a tendency to move in another direction. For instance, if a therapist is not comfortable with anger, or that therapist has his or her own issues around sexual abuse, he or she may have difficulty allowing the client to experience the full range of emotions that accompanies those topics.

This is not usually a purposeful act by the therapist but instead a quite normal reaction to distress. If you sense that your therapist may be uncomfortable around a particular subject, or you experience the therapist steering you away from talking about something of importance to you, bring it up. The really good therapist will be receptive to your feedback and will consider what you are relating to him or her.

Too Aloof or Too Chatty

Small talk is the more common way for two people who haven't seen each other in a while to break the ice. Whether you are working out at the gym or getting ready to delve into your therapy, warming up can be a helpful way to build momentum. Some therapists may not recognize when you are relying on them to take the work deeper, instead remaining too long with superficial banter. Because therapy sessions tend to be approximately forty-five minutes long, which occupies a very small portion of your week, it is important to make the most of your time.

As the therapy relationship progresses, small talk may increase or decrease, depending upon the relationship. For instance, at the start of therapy, it may be all business, or it may be a slow buildup to core issues. Once the relationship is established, it may feel like a friendship, and you may want to talk about extraneous issues with the therapist. Some therapists are very eager to talk about world events or unrelated matters. Exchanging recipes, predictions about football games, and discussion of current events are all innocuous if done proportionally.

Taking Sides (Couples Therapy)

No matter how experienced a therapist is, he or she is going to have opinions about each partner, maybe even judgments they haven't yet looked inward to understand. As a trained observer of relationships, the therapist's job is to assess the mechanics of a relationship and help each partner raise his or her awareness of what he or she is doing to influence the process of relatedness.

At times a therapist may feel very strongly about the behavior of one person, in particular when one of the clients seems oppressed or overpowered. In these instances, temptation to gravitate toward one partner may grow. The outcome can be harmful to the relationship because the imbalance of support can lead to greater resentment on one side and further disempowerment on the other.

Keep in mind this is not to imply that therapists don't focus on one person or another during part of the session. What I am describing is a prolonged and obvious departure from the objective stance into an alignment with one person. This may be either overt or not obvious, depending upon the situation. If you feel as though your therapist is not seeing both sides or has aligned with one person, you can make the therapist aware of this. Too many clients leave therapy prematurely because they experience this very event and give up too quickly. Couples therapy is not about making one person right and one person wrong. If one person is "wrong," then both partners lose.

Giving Too Much Advice

Therapy is not about telling people what to do. Although therapists can be construed as experts on human behavior, they are not the expert on you. Nobody knows better what to do than you, and if you feel lost or stuck, then look for a therapist to help you figure this out as opposed to directing you toward their answer. If your therapist continues saying what you should be doing, reliance on that therapist is generated instead of self-reliance, which is the ultimate goal of therapy.

Advising may be a part of therapy in certain instances. Therapists routinely give their opinions or provide you with feedback about how they view your circumstance. Oftentimes this advice is intended to help you become stronger while you are doing the work of therapy, such as suggesting how working out at a gym may help you burn stress and build stamina. Sometimes advice takes the form of suggesting coping mechanisms, such as journaling or creating a schedule. These are simple examples of advice that does not foster dependence.

If the larger issues you are dealing with in therapy lead to advice giving from your therapist, then you may have cause for concern. Advice tends to be the most impersonal and ineffective form of support. Even in your personal life, advice is a way of not getting intimate with whomever you are dealing with, because all you are lending is your thoughts or beliefs, based on your own subjective experience.

If this happens, bringing it to the attention of the therapist, no matter how tempting it is to take his or her direction, can help you take greater ownership of your work. Listening to your therapist's advice can have two likely outcomes—you are successful, in which case the credit goes to them (and you can't feel as good about it), or it turns out poorly and you have somebody else to hold responsible. Neither is a helpful option for long-term growth.

Insufficient Feedback

Many clients come into therapy with some notion of what the experience will be like. This idea is derived from stories, movies, books, general fantasy, and any prior experience they may have had. One of the biggest myths for first-time clients is that therapists don't say much during a session, but instead just ponder their thoughts while smoking a pipe and rubbing their chin saying, "Hmmm."

This would hardly be helpful to anybody who needs more than a warm body in the room to talk at. Instead, therapy is about an open exchange of ideas, where beliefs can be expanded, thinking broadened, and emotions expressed. Unfortunately, some therapists do not recognize that a client needs more than is being given, and clients are often reluctant to make this need known.

Therapists may not provide sufficient feedback for several reasons, none of which will become known without you, as the client, speaking up. The possibilities may include caution due to not knowing you well enough (therapists have to feel safe with you as well), not knowing you wanted to hear more, a therapy style in which the clinician doesn't offer as much as you want, and a desire not to influence you, to name a few.

It is important, particularly early in your relationship building, that you let the therapist know if you are not getting enough input from him or her. This is perfectly alright to ask for, and the therapist may be grateful for the direction.

Being Too Much of an "Expert"

We tend to feel the best when we are in control of the work we do in therapy. If we come to some important realization or implement a successful experiment, the reward is greater if it was self-generated. This is not to say the therapist ought not be involved with the creative process; it means that the more ownership we as clients have over the design and implementation, the better we feel. This holds true for teaching children as well.

If the therapist you are working with comes off as too much of an expert, that therapist may do so for their own self-interest of feeling important, as opposed to your well-being. This can be a hindrance to therapy because the therapist may not be as receptive to your feedback, or the therapist may not allow you to be in charge of your therapy.

While we want therapists to be knowledgeable and even have expertise about our predicaments, we don't want them to be the expert of us. This is a frequent reason for clients to become disenfranchised with therapy, because the power dynamics in the relationship seem imbalanced. Know-it-alls are generally turnoffs in our lives, and the same applies to therapists.

Taking Too Much or Too Little Responsibility

Who is ultimately responsible for the success of your therapy? Some might argue it is the client; after all, the clients are the ones who determine how hard they work and how much risk taking they are willing to do. Others might say it is the therapist, because they are guiding the process. The answer lies somewhere in the middle, as it does with any relationship. A therapist who feels too responsible for a client's success can put too much pressure on the client. A therapist who takes too little responsibility can leave a client feeling as though the therapist isn't invested enough, which leaves that client feeling too much on his or her own.

A client should never feel blamed by their therapist for not working hard enough or not making gains. It's quite alright for a therapist to confront a client or point out to them where they believe being stuck comes from, but putting it squarely on the shoulders of the client will likely lead to greater stuck-ness.

Not Recognizing Our Own "Stuff"

There is ongoing debate in the therapeutic community regarding the role of the therapist and how authentic one ought to be. This means that some clinicians believe they are there to be neutral and objective figures, allowing clients to project feelings onto them for interpretation. Others believe that therapists ought to be more human and genuine, sharing openly how they are experiencing their client, including what feelings are generated for them throughout the course of a session.

There is no correct answer in general, but there can certainly be a right answer for working with you. Just because a clinician has a feeling about or toward his or her client does not mean that feeling should be shared. Sometimes what a client brings up to the therapist in a therapy session has little to do with the client but is instead about the therapist's own life.

Therapists make a mistake by being unaware of the thoughts and feelings that are sparked for them during the course of therapy. If thera-

pists are not aware of what gets stirred from within, they may inadvertently allow it to influence the work with their clients. If the therapist is aware
of what is being triggered for them, they have the option of addressing it
openly or on their own, but at least it will be less likely to impede their
work if it's known to them.

There is no cause for alarm, because this happens *all the time*. A
therapist reacts spontaneously to a client, so the potential is high for a
therapist to make a statement to a client that is generated by something
unrelated. As a client, you may not be aware when this happens, but there
is a way to check it out. If you find that feedback you are given does not
make sense to you or fit with your gut instinct, you can ask the therapist
about it. Many therapists welcome the opportunity to consider and talk
about themselves—it's a result of being present for others much of their
day.

Not Challenging or Confronting Complacency

Therapy is about supporting, encouraging, and stimulating insight and
awareness. In doing this we generate momentum toward change or acceptance. When inertia sets in for clients who find it difficult to generate self-
initiative, it is the therapist's job to help those clients understand their
resistance to change. Beyond this promotion of self-understanding, it is
also the job of the therapist to help clients take action to get their needs
met, which doesn't always happen through the tactics described above.
Sometimes the movement is more like a car that is trapped in the snow;
the car needs to be rocked back and forth until traction can be gained. The
rocking also allows clients to feel both ends of a continuum, helpful
before deciding on a path.

Therapists may not want to push their clients beyond their comfort
levels out of fear, respect, or a belief this will not be helpful. This may be
accurate if clients feel too fragile or their situation is overly chaotic. At
such times a client can feel trapped or unwelcoming of such prompting,
or the discomfort may even serve to strengthen that client's resistance,
alienating him or her from the therapist.

In some cases, however, a gentle shove is exactly what's needed to
create movement. As the client, it is important that you provide your
therapist with feedback on what degree of prompting you can handle, or if
you are getting too little or too much prompting. Pointing out when

somebody's body isn't matching their words, or their thoughts seem contrary to their needs, are examples of gentle pushing. Other examples may include more direct challenge of inertia that is still kind and compassionate.

Not Meeting Clients Where They Are

When clients initially come into therapy, they have varying degrees of understanding about their situations and what needs to happen to get to where they need to be. They have differing levels of understanding about the nature of therapy and how it can be used to accomplish one's goals. Because of this, no prescriptive treatment works for everyone. Instead, therapy must be custom tailored to each individual. We use the term *meeting clients where they are* to describe this assessment process to help determine where help is needed.

The creative process in therapy means adaptability to and cognizance of where a person begins their work. If somebody is highly guarded and skeptical of therapy, fearful of their privacy, engaging in safe discussions may be best. If it's a teenager who is put off by the clinical setting of your office, taking a walk outside may help. The bottom line is meeting the client as opposed to trying to lasso and drag them toward your position.

Not Addressing the Therapeutic Relationship

The relationship between client and therapist is, in many ways, similar to any other relationship. There is a need for trust, openness, and honesty, and shared experiences unite and separate the pair. This professional-personal relationship is finite, however, in that there will be a time when the relationship comes to a close, if only for a portion of time. Even though the relationship may seem clearly imbalanced, there will still be a time to explore the dynamics within.

Even though therapy is all about the client, meaning no negotiation around reciprocity or an exchange of needs, there are times that both may feel let down, diminished, taken for granted, and so on.

If the therapist and the client don't tend to their relationship, several problems may emerge. First, the client needs to know when and if they are being judged. Words may also be spoken by the therapist that evoke uncomfortable emotions, even resentment at times. Without periodic check-ins, rifts may develop, ultimately sabotaging the work of the client.

It is also good practice to talk about the relationship. In our everyday lives we tend to avoid direct conversations about our experience of others, instead choosing to use conduits and go-betweens. Speaking with your therapist about how you experience them, either warmly or contrarily, can provide the practice needed to navigate those very important relationships in your life.

Ignoring Issues of Diversity (Gender, Sexuality, Ethnicity, etc.)

Unless you are seeing a therapist who is an exact replica of yourself, which can be limiting, differences are likely to exist. The most noticeable dissimilarities are those of race, gender, and ethnicity, although many others are less apparent. When screening a therapist for the first time, you may want to find one who shares certain value systems, such as religious beliefs, but for some people this is not a priority. At some point in the therapy, this may be an important topic to discuss because it can produce tension.

It is advisable for therapists to address these potential influences on therapy early on so that clients can be teachers for the therapist. That is, clients teach therapists about who they are, including their traditions, values, and the beliefs that influence them throughout their lives. In this way, therapists can gain a broader perspective of who their clients are and how they might be useful in helping them address their goals. Most importantly, addressing differences can help to prevent offending or disrespecting.

Poor Boundaries (Being Your Friend)

The description "poor boundaries" may not be the best terminology, but it's the most recognizable. Boundaries are actually points of contact, ways of defining ourselves to help us relate with others. When boundaries aren't clearly defined or the distinction between personal and professional is blurred, problems may arise.

Many clients want to feel cared for, and some may even wish the relationship would not involve a business component. The exchange of money and use of a contract may be viewed as unfortunate by clients who feel close to their therapist, wishing for a relationship like this in their lives. The responsible professional will recognize this and address the matter as a learning opportunity, rather than simply meeting the needs of the client. While the instinct to be friends with one's client may seem innocuous, it can cause confusion and even considerable harm to the client.

Once that professional relationship crosses over into a more personal relationship, the potential for problems will grow. There are therapists who subscribe to orientations that don't maintain such rigid boundaries, allowing for the expression of warm or even unpleasant feelings between the two; however, this is often part of the therapy process. There are also therapists who may attend a wedding or funeral of a long-term client, which is generally the case when a very solid relationship has been established where such an occurrence would be well thought out.

RESISTANCE TO CHANGE

Resistance is defined in the dictionary as confrontation or opposition. Resistance is viewed as synonymous with battle, struggle, fight, or any such type of confrontation. Interestingly enough, the antonym given for resistance is *surrender*, meaning that victory is the goal in dealing with resistance. So if one uses this definition to conceptualize resistance, we come away with the idea that those who display resistance are a threat to those in power. The way to deal with this threat must then involve overpowering, coercion, or perhaps avoidance. Let's first look at how resistance works within a person and then compare it to the process of negotiation between people.

Consider the muscles in your shoulders and neck. If you want to let go and relax, your head will slump forward (if you are sitting upright). If you are sitting in a chair and your head is not slumped forward, your body is resisting the option for too much relaxation. You were not paying attention to this resistance to letting go of your neck muscles, yet it was constantly there. Consider as well your energy level and the degree of fatigue in your body. You may be tired and want to close your eyes, but instead you are keeping them open to read this book. These examples represent the very physical intrapersonal (within body) conflict that keeps your momentum paced in such a way that change does not occur too quickly.

This conflict also occurs between people. In another example, you may feel conflicted about something or somebody in your life, and you are choosing whether or not to intervene in some way. Perhaps you are unhappy with your job or a relationship in your life but have decided to wait it out instead of making a change. These are all examples of conflicts taking place within the body at various levels—physiological, emotional, and cognitive—all of which create uncertainty in one's life.

The conflict that helps regulate the process of change is also known as resistance. Resistance creates a constant tension state within the body that helps mobilize us to take action toward getting our needs met. If the tension is too low, we become flat and unresponsive, otherwise known as depression. If the tension is too high, we become hypervigilant and "stressed out," exhausted mentally and physically.

The optimal level of tension is a balancing act that requires regular attention. This balancing act is analogous to a fisherman who lets out a certain amount of line so a fish can take the bait. If there is too much slack in the line, the fisherman may not know the fish is present and the bait may be taken before a response is made. If the line is too taut, the fish may be scared away by impulsive jerking of the rod.

The maintenance of our tension states is a process that occurs largely beyond our awareness. We are not concentrating as intently as the fisherman because there are so many choice points in our life, so many conflicts that emerge through the course of a day, that we go on autopilot to reach our destination. We forget the importance of how we are getting to where we would like to be and simply focus on the end result. We are not recognizing how much uncertainty exists in our lives, in part because acknowledging this may lead us to feeling out of control. So instead we pretend not to notice our ambivalence and function as if we have it all together. Although change is going on all the time, we attempt to steer this change in a certain direction.

Imagine a married couple who are largely unaware of how they navigate resistance. Whenever absolute agreement is not found, some form of battle will take place, with one person being victorious and the other wounded by defeat. Depending on what style of adaptation is used to deal with the resistance, the loser may feel overpowered, manipulated, or disregarded. Consequently, the winner may feel defeated as well, since the loser of this particular dispute will find a way of repaying his or her partner with passivity, withdrawal, or another form of retaliation.

If this style of interaction continues over any sustained period of time, a number of results will be likely. Within the relationship, there will be a loss of intimacy due to the distance created by the win-lose outcome of conflicts. A power differential will likely be established that alters the communication style of the couple so that covert operations replace a more open and honest mode of interaction.

For each individual within the dyad, a different phenomenon can be found. The one who typically comes out on top of conflicts learns this is the preferred mode of relating and utilizes this style in other circumstances. He or she learns to seek out others who can be overpowered and will submit to those with more authority. A survival-of-the-fittest mentality ensues that creates hierarchical patterns within their system. Loneliness is often times the result, as genuine relating with vulnerability and receptivity is lost.

Conversely, the individual who more frequently comes out on the bottom of conflict experiences the situation quite differently. Symptoms such as anxiety and depression are present, as these people have learned that helplessness is inevitable. The person may feel it no longer matters what he or she does, because there will not be a chance of success. This loss of power can also lead to a loss of genuine contact with others due to his or her victim mentality.

The balance-oriented orientation assumes that there is a great deal of ambivalence regarding change in any system (individual or organizational). The difference is this approach views ambivalence as normal, potentially useful, and oftentimes valuable. If we can become curious about this ambivalence such that we explore it at a deeper level, the nature of the resistance can be better understood. In fact, once we understand the underlying meaning of the resistance, we can find protective, curative, and creative aspects of resistance to utilize. Our task is to find ways to harness this energy appropriately to get our needs met.

As difficult as it may seem to be curious about resistance (as it may be considered a threat), consider it an experiment in relating. You need not use this approach if it doesn't fit with your style of leading, but for the time being, leave the window partly open just in case you find some idea that resonates with your approach. As you read the proceeding pages it is important to continuously pay attention to your own experience of resistance. When concepts do not fit within your schema of understanding, recognize this lack of fit and pay attention to what you do with it. Do you disregard the idea as silly or stupid? Do you minimize the importance of what is being suggested as if you had not read it? Or, perhaps, do you pretend to understand what is being offered but in actuality cannot make sense of it?

WHAT MAKES SOMEBODY SUCCESSFUL IN THERAPY

- Self-awareness
- Receptiveness to feedback
- Risk taking/experimentation
- Persistence
- Challenging the therapist
- Resources
- Willingness to experience

Self-Awareness

Self-awareness is the ability to see oneself clearly in relation to others. If I know that I am stubborn and that others experience me this way, making it difficult for them to negotiate with me, then I will have a better chance of working on this quality.

A person does not need to enter therapy being self-aware, but if they work toward curiosity about how others see them in order to better understand themselves, they will be better positioned to grow.

Those who lack self-awareness can compensate by being incredibly interested in how others see them, soliciting feedback whenever possible. Learning to scan one's internal and external environments, meaning to examine what is going on inside us and between us and another person, will also help with this task.

Receptiveness to Feedback

Even if input from a therapist is contrary to how you see yourself, or unpleasant to hear, the more willing you are to take in feedback the more likely you are to grow.

People who enter group therapy, which is a very scary medium for newcomers to therapy but among the most powerful venues for personal growth, are the most likely to improve in this way. The seasoned group therapy client will learn to seek out feedback every chance they get, become excited by the prospect of somebody reacting to them (even aversive), and strive to incorporate this information into their learning.

On the contrary, we don't want to be so impressionable that everything told to us is accepted without chewing on it. Being receptive to input does not mean being a sponge without filters, as this would turn us into clay, changing shape every time somebody talks to us.

Risk Taking/Experimentation

Risk taking means leaning into discomfort. The terms can be synonymous, as they both mean going toward the sound of the cannon. When we sense discomfort, we know learning is on the horizon. Not much changes without some degree of unpleasantness, so continue improving your tolerance of distress so that you can venture into the unknown.

Our dark sides, or the parts of ourselves we are least comfortable sharing with others, largely because we fear it will result in rejection, requires continuous seeking out. Engaging with people in new ways, through conflict and intimacy; altering the way we talk to ourselves; listening to new parts of our being; and seeking challenges in our personal and professional life will result in new growth.

Experiments are calculated risks based on new hypotheses. If we discover that we don't confront others because we fear it will result in rejection, an experiment would be some testing of this theory. We generally do a good bit of work trying to understand the possible results of this risk so that we are prepared for different outcomes. If we can place the value of taking risks over the outcomes, we are generally ready to do this work.

Persistence

Nothing worthwhile comes easily. This is a motto worth living by for those engaged in any type of personal growth work. If we are going to be exuberant about the result of our efforts in therapy, we want to be prepared for the likelihood that constant roadblocks and pitfalls will be in our path.

Therapy and personal growth work can feel like trekking through sludge with a hundred-pound weight on your back, oftentimes in the dark and cold. With everything working against you at times, including health, financial stress, childcare issues, work stress, and general malaise, know that your journey will be fraught with challenges.

If you push yourself even at the times when you feel your worst and remain loyal to your process, good things will happen. In group therapy this never seems to be more true. Those who consider ending group work for a multitude of reasons generally find that important learning is waiting for them when they overcome their resistance.

Challenging the Therapist

For somebody doing their personal growth work in therapy, there will come a time, and many of them, when you will need to confront your therapist. You will be dissatisfied, angry, upset, hurt by, and generally disgusted with your therapist if you work with them long enough. No matter how skilled or caring your therapist is, they are human. In order for the relationship to thrive, you will need to tell them when you are displeased.

Telling your therapist you were unhappy with something they said, did, didn't say, or didn't do doesn't mean they were wrong. If we get away from the idea that a perfect exists, we will explore this type of unpleasantness in a way that will both support our own learning and strengthen the bond with the therapist.

If your therapist is too passive, too challenging, seeming bored, missing appointments, frequently late, uninspired, or off putting in any number of ways, consider telling them how you feel. Any therapist worth seeing will be receptive to your feedback. Expect some level of resistance or dialogue to ensue, but make sure they take in your feelings. Even if your experience is based on your own "stuff," the only way to get to this is to feel heard and understood.

Resources

On a more pragmatic level, having people in your corner will make your journey more productive. You need them to hold you accountable, encourage you, serve as a mirror, bounce ideas off, disclose to, practice with, and generally be in your corner.

If you don't have a good support system, this is a worthwhile early goal to work on. If your personal growth work involves any type of significant work, it is imperative that you have people to support you when you get stuck.

Willingness to Experience

If you are working with a therapist who is not solely focused on your thinking, you will learn how to access parts of yourself that are less active. For most people in the Western hemisphere, this means learning how to listen to our bodies. In doing so, we can access our sensations, feelings, needs, and experiences, beginning the process of reintegration.

Becoming whole or fully integrated means learning how to access those pieces that we have distanced ourselves from, whether they be memories, instincts, fantasies, drives, impulses, feelings, and so on, that seem undesirable.

Therapy and personal growth work will more likely be a transformative experience if we allow ourselves to go in this direction.

Appendix

GLOSSARY OF TERMS AND THEIR DEFINITIONS

Clinician *Clinician* is a term interchangeable with *psychotherapist.*

Counselor *Counselor* is a generic term sometimes interchangeable with *therapist* or *clinician.* Counselors generally get their master's degree, but many have only a bachelor's degree. There are national exams for counselors, including the NBCC (Nationally Board Certified Counselor). Counselors can also attain state licenses, such as the LPC (Licensed Professional Counselor) in New Jersey and Pennsylvania. LPCs are eligible to work with managed care/insurance companies.

Life coach A life coach is somebody who works on specific objectives that do not require in-depth analysis or investigation. This is a relatively new specialty, and training programs and certificates are available.

Patient versus client Depending upon the length of time a therapist has been in practice and their philosophical orientation, these terms are used interchangeably.

Psychologist A psychologist has completed four years of college and at least four years of a doctoral program in clinical, counseling, school, industrial, or other. In addition, he or she has passed a national test and fulfilled the state requirements specific to that region. A psychologist may either be a Psy.D. (doctor of psychology) or Ph.D. (doctor of philosophy). There is little difference in the programs except that Psy.D. is a newer degree and is less heavily research based. Psychologists are eligible to work with managed care/insurance companies. Psychologists who specialize in psychotherapy and other forms of psychological treatment are highly trained professionals with expertise in behavior, mental health assessment, diagnosis and treatment, and behavior change.

Psychotherapist A psychotherapist is a particular type of therapist who works with emotional, behavioral, and psychological issues. There are certifications but no licenses for this type of practitioner. Psychotherapists apply scientifically validated procedures to help people change their thoughts, emotions, and behaviors. Psychotherapy is a collaborative effort between an individual and a psychotherapist. It provides a supportive environment to talk openly and confidentially about concerns and feelings. Psychotherapists consider client confidentiality extremely important and will answer questions regarding those rare circumstances when confidential information must be shared.

Social worker Social workers can be LSWs or LCSWs, depending upon their licensure. LCSWs have accumulated sufficient hours of supervision and have passed a test by the Social Work Board. All social workers get their master's degree from a specialized training program. Only LCSWs are invited to participate with managed care/insurance companies. An MSW may also be a therapist, but they are not licensed and have different restrictions.

Therapist Anybody can call themselves a therapist, and the focus of their work can include many areas, including physical, occupational, spiritual, mental health, and so on.

NOTES

INTRODUCTION

1. "Psychology Today," last modified April 29, 2014, http://www.camft.org/ScriptContent/CAMFTarticles/Misc/TherapyInAmerica.htm.

1. WHAT IS (PSYCHO) THERAPY?

1. Alex Kotlowitz (1991). *There Are No Children Here: The Story of Two Boys Growing Up in the Other America.* New York: Anchor Books.
2. Charles Bates (1991). *Pigs Eat Wolves: Going into Partnership with Your Dark Side.* St. Paul, MN: Yes International Publisher.
3. Carl Rogers (1965). *Client-Centered Therapy.* Boston: Houghton Mifflin Company.
4. Carl Rogers (1965). *Client-Centered Therapy.* Boston: Houghton Mifflin Company.
5. Ann Olson, "Theory and Psychopathology," *Psychology Today* http://www.psychologytoday.com/blog/theory-and-psychopathology/201308/the-theory-self-actualization.
6. "NIMH," 2014, http://www.nimh.nih.gov/statistics/SMI_AASR.shtml.
7. "APA," 2012, http://www.apa.org/news/press/releases/2012/09/psychotherapy.aspx.
8. "APA," 2012, https://www.apa.org/. http://www.apa.org/news/press/releases/2012/09/psychotherapy.aspx.
9. http://www.apa.org/monitor/2013/01/depression.aspx.

10. "NAMI," 2014, http://www.nami.org/template.cfm?section=about_ mental_illness.

2. HOW DOES THERAPY WORK?

1. Carol Gilligan (1982). *In a Different Voice: Psychological Theory and Women's Development*. Cambridge, MA: Harvard University Press.

3. WHY DO PEOPLE GO TO THERAPY?

1. "National Institute of Mental Health," last modified June 19, 2014,http:// www.nimh.nih.gov/index.shtml.

2. "SAMHSA," last modified June 19, 2014, http://www.namigc.org/wp-content/uploads/2013/01/MentalIllnessFactSheet-July-2013.pdf.

3. "NAMI," last modified June 19, 2014, http://www.nami.org/template. cfm?section=about_mental_illness.

4. "NAMI," last modified June 19, 2014, http://www.nami.org/template. cfm?section=about_mental_illness.

5. "NAMI," last modified June 19, 2014, http://www.nami.org/template. cfm?section=about_mental_illness.

6. "NAMI," last modified June 19, 2014, http://www.nami.org/template. cfm?section=about_mental_illness.

7. "ADAA," last modified June 19, 2014, http://www.adaa.org/about-adaa/ press-room/facts-statistics.

8. "ADAA," last modified June 19, 2014, http://www.adaa.org/about-adaa/ press-room/facts-statistics.

9. "ADAA," last modified June 19, 2014, http://www.adaa.org/about-adaa/ press-room/facts-statistics.

10. "ADAA," last modified June 19, 2014, http://www.adaa.org/about-adaa/ press-room/facts-statistics.

11. "ADAA," last modified June 19, 2014, http://www.adaa.org/about-adaa/ press-room/facts-statistics.

12. "National Institute of Mental Health," last modified June 19, 2014, http:// www.nimh.nih.gov/index.shtml.

13. "National Institute of Mental Health," last modified June 19, 2014, http:// www.nimh.nih.gov/index.shtml.

14. "National Institute of Mental Health," last modified June 19, 2014, http:// www.nimh.nih.gov/index.shtml.

15. "National Institute of Mental Health," last modified June 19, 2014, http://www.nimh.nih.gov/index.shtml.

16. "National Institute of Mental Health," last modified June 19, 2014, http://www.nimh.nih.gov/index.shtml.

17. "National Institute of Mental Health," last modified June 19, 2014, http://www.nimh.nih.gov/index.shtml.

18. "National Institute of Mental Health," last modified June 19, 2014, http://www.nimh.nih.gov/index.shtml.

19. "World Health Organization," last modified June 19, 2014, http://www.who.int/whr/2001/media_centre/en/whr01_fact_sheet1_en.pdf.

20. "National Institute of Mental Health," last modified June 19, 2014, http://www.nimh.nih.gov/index.shtml.

21. "National Institute of Mental Health," last modified June 19, 2014, http://www.nimh.nih.gov/index.shtml.

22. "National Institute of Mental Health," last modified June 19, 2014, http://www.nimh.nih.gov/index.shtml.

23. "National Institute of Mental Health," last modified June 19, 2014, http://www.nimh.nih.gov/index.shtml.

24. "National Institute of Mental Health," last modified June 19, 2014, http://www.nimh.nih.gov/index.shtml.

25. "National Institute of Mental Health," last modified June 19, 2014, http://www.nimh.nih.gov/index.shtml.

26. "National Institute of Mental Health," last modified June 19, 2014,http://www.nimh.nih.gov/index.shtml.

27. "American Viewpoint Survey," last modified June 19, 2014, http://www.nationaleatingdisorders.org/get-facts-eating-disorders.

28. "American Viewpoint Survey," last modified June 19, 2014, http://www.nationaleatingdisorders.org/get-facts-eating-disorders.

29. "American Viewpoint Survey," last modified June 19, 2014, http://www.nationaleatingdisorders.org/get-facts-eating-disorders.

30. "American Viewpoint Survey," last modified June 19, 2014, http://www.nationaleatingdisorders.org/get-facts-eating-disorders.

31. "American Viewpoint Survey," last modified June 19, 2014, http://www.nationaleatingdisorders.org/get-facts-eating-disorders.

32. "National Institute of Mental Health," last modified June 19, 2014, http://www.nimh.nih.gov/index.shtml.

33. "National Institute of Mental Health," last modified June 19, 2014, http://www.nimh.nih.gov/index.shtml.

34. "Business Insider.com," last retrieved June 19, 2014, http://www.businessinsider.com/what-do-you-do-when-you-hate-your-job-2010-10#!HG8SR.

5. THEORETICAL ORIENTATION

1. James Kepner (1996). *Healing Tasks: Psychotherapy with Adult Survivors of Childhood Abuse*. The Analytic Press.

6. UNDERSTANDING MANAGED CARE AND HEALTH INSURANCE

1. "NAMI," last modified June 23, 2014, http://www.nami.org/factsheets/mentalillness_factsheet.pdf.
2. "NAMI," last modified June 23, 2014, http://www.nami.org/factsheets/mentalillness_factsheet.pdf.
3. "NAMI," last modified June 23, 2014, http://www.nami.org/factsheets/mentalillness_factsheet.pdf.
4. "NAMI," last modified June 23, 2014, http://www.nami.org/factsheets/mentalillness_factsheet.pdf.

7. PATIENT RIGHTS AND RESPONSIBILITIES

1. World Psychiatry, 2011; "NCBI," last retrieved on June 23, 2014, http://www.ncbi.nlm.nih.gov/pmc/articles/PMC3104888/.
2. "NAMI," last retrieved on June 23, 2014, http://www.nami.org/factsheets/mentalillness_factsheet.pdf.
3. "NAMI," last retrieved on June 23, 2014, http://www.nami.org/factsheets/mentalillness_factsheet.pdf.
4. "NAMI," last retrieved on June 23, 2014, http://www.nami.org/factsheets/mentalillness_factsheet.pdf.

9. THE FIRST FEW SESSIONS

1. Michael Craig Clemmens (2005). *Getting Beyond Sobriety: Clinical Approaches to Long-Term Recovery*. New York: Gestalt Press.

10. THERAPY CONCENTRATION AREAS

1. "APA," 2014, https://www.apa.org/helpcenter/eating.aspx.

2. "APA," 2014, https://www.apa.org/helpcenter/eating.aspx.

3. "Medicine Net," 2014, http://www.medicinenet.com/depression/article. htm#depression_facts.

4. "Medicine Net," 2014, http://www.medicinenet.com/depression/article. htm#depression_facts.

5. "Medicine Net," 2014, http://www.medicinenet.com/depression/article. htm#depression_facts.

11. A WHOLISTIC APPROACH TO WELLNESS

1. "NAMI," 2014, http://www.nami.org/Content/NavigationMenu/Inform_ Yourself/About_Mental_Illness/About_Mental_Illness.htm.

2. "NAMI," 2014, http://www.nami.org/Content/NavigationMenu/Inform_ Yourself/About_Mental_Illness/About_Mental_Illness.htm.

3. "NAMI," 2014, http://www.nami.org/Content/NavigationMenu/Inform_ Yourself/About_Mental_Illness/About_Mental_Illness.htm.

4. APA, *Coping with Serious Illness*, https://www.apa.org/topics/stress/ index.aspx.

5. APA, *Learned Optimism Yields Health Benefits*, https://www.apa.org/ pubs/index.aspx.

6. APA, *Coping with Serious Illness*, https://www.apa.org/topics/stress/ index.aspx.

7. APA, *Coping with Serious Illness*, https://www.apa.org/topics/stress/ index.aspx.

8. APA, *Coping with Serious Illness*, https://www.apa.org/topics/stress/ index.aspx.

12. ALTERNATIVE HEALTH CARE

1. Joel Fuhrman (2011). *Super Immunity: The Essential Nutrition Guide for Boosting Your Body's Defenses to Live Longer, Stronger, and Disease Free.* New York: Harper Collins Publishers.

2. "NIM," last retrieved on June 23, 2014, http://report.nih.gov/ nihfactsheets/viewfactsheet.aspx?csid=102.

3. "NIM," last retrieved on June 23, 2014, http://report.nih.gov/ nihfactsheets/viewfactsheet.aspx?csid=102.

4. "NIM," last retrieved on June 23, 2014, http://report.nih.gov/ nihfactsheets/viewfactsheet.aspx?csid=102.

5. "CNN," last retrieved on 06-23-2014, http://www.cnn.com/2014/02/04/health/who-world-cancer-report/.

6. "NIM," last retrieved on June 23, 2014, http://report.nih.gov/nihfactsheets/viewfactsheet.aspx?csid=102.

7. "NIM," last retrieved on June 23, 2014, http://report.nih.gov/nihfactsheets/viewfactsheet.aspx?csid=102.

8. "NIM," last retrieved on June 23, 2014, http://report.nih.gov/nihfactsheets/viewfactsheet.aspx?csid=102.

9. "NIM," last retrieved on June 23, 2014, http://report.nih.gov/nihfactsheets/viewfactsheet.aspx?csid=102.

10. "NIM," last retrieved on June 23, 2014, http://report.nih.gov/nihfactsheets/viewfactsheet.aspx?csid=102.

11. "NIM," last retrieved on June 23, 2014, http://report.nih.gov/nihfactsheets/viewfactsheet.aspx?csid=102.

INDEX